building breakthroughs

Raju Prasad

building breakthroughs

On the Frontier of Medical Innovation

 Johns Hopkins University Press Baltimore

© 2022 Johns Hopkins University Press
All rights reserved. Published 2022
Printed in the United States of America on acid-free paper
9 8 7 6 5 4 3 2 1

Johns Hopkins University Press
2715 North Charles Street
Baltimore, Maryland 21218-4363
www.press.jhu.edu

Library of Congress Cataloging-in-Publication Data is available.

ISBN-13: 978-1-4214-4487-1 (hardcover)
ISBN-13: 978-1-4214-4488-8 (electronic)

A catalog record for this book is available from the British Library.

*Special discounts are available for bulk purchases of this book. For more information,
please contact Special Sales at specialsales@jh.edu.*

For Maya and Neela—

Always believe in yourselves and each other

and

To the memory of Dr. M. G. Prasad—

"Learning has a beginning but no end"

Contents

part II
Enabling the Next Wave of Innovation

Contents

viii

building breakthroughs

Introduction

With our ever-increasing understanding of biology, as well as technological advances that are enabling the accrual and analysis of large quantities of data, we are reaching a tipping point for medical breakthroughs. The types of discoveries that regularly populate the pages of journals such as *Science, Nature,* and the *New England Journal of Medicine* are elucidating more and more complex and elegant mechanisms of how the human body works and how we might act to meaningfully ameliorate or even eradicate diseases. The expansive foundation of knowledge developed in biology leads many to believe it has the potential to become the "new tech" over the next decade.[1] In his 2016 State of the Union address, President Barack Obama asked the nation, "How do we reignite that spirit of innovation to meet our biggest challenges?" and announced the Cancer Moonshot, an initiative with the goal of making "America the country that cures cancer once and for all."[2]

When President John F. Kennedy delivered his vision for a moonshot before a joint session of Congress on May 25, 1961, he set a clear goal: "I believe that this nation should commit itself to achieving the goal, before this decade is out, of landing a man on the moon and returning him safely to the earth. No single space project in this period will be more impressive to mankind, or more important for the long-range exploration of space; and none will be so difficult or expensive to accomplish."[3] Since the successful Apollo 11 landing on July 20, 1969, the word "moonshot" has been used across disciplines. It is broadly defined as an a priori plan to boldly approach a problem. In contrast, a "breakthrough" is a gradual improvement in a field until a solution to a problem is found through an alternative approach or, perhaps, by serendipity or luck. In biotechnology and medicine, the term "breakthrough" is more apt for recent discoveries, given the sometimes laborious clinical and regulatory elements that make the process of innovation more iterative (it is sometimes referred to as "linear innovation") than its technology counterpart.

The central focus of this book is to explore examples of medical breakthroughs, going from a patient's diagnosis, to an idea, to the development of the therapeutic, and, finally, regulatory approval. I then discuss what has been learned from the development of these therapies, or "building blocks," that can help continue the wave of innovation. In 2020, the world saw these processes play out in real time on the global stage with each aspect of the development of COVID-19 therapeutics and vaccines. What became glaringly clear was that the communication and "demystification" of drug development from lab bench to bedside could not be more necessary.

In part I of this book, I start with the journey of individual patients, profiling people who had a disease that progressed to a point where it was untreatable by the standard therapies at that time. I look at challenges that face patients with leukemia and lymphoma, as well as the rare disorders of spinal muscular atrophy (SMA) and sickle cell anemia. I then discuss the development of selected breakthroughs in medicine, progressing from an idea to their path to gain approval. I dive into the stories behind three examples of medical breakthroughs developed in recent years. Their remarkable results, in my view, signal the beginning of a genomic revolution in the treatment of diseases:

1. Therapies that utilize a patient's own immune cells, reprogramming them to target cancerous cells (for leukemia and lymphoma), thus creating a type of living medicine.
2. A method to deliver a copy of a gene into a patient with a mutation in that very gene (for SMA).
3. A way to reprogram stem cells in the blood to counteract the effects of a devastating genetic blood disorder (for sickle cell anemia).

Each of these therapies presents awe-inspiring improvements offering real benefits to patients and represents the promise of using cell and gene therapies to treat disease. Such breakthroughs highlight perseverance and science's ability to build on prior knowledge, collaboration as well as competition, an increasing ability to leverage technology in support of health care, an "ecosystem," or environment that enables experimentation (and must continue to do so), an acceptance of failure, and the gumption to change course.

While these are tried-and-true concepts, the next wave of innovation in biotechnology may also come from those focused on big ideas, such as correcting one or several mutations in DNA among the 3 billion sequences in the human genome; identifying populations at risk of serious diseases earlier than ever before; and understanding and treating cancerous tumors in a targeted manner, to avoid the side effects of chemotherapy. Indeed, the growth of our technological capacity has the potential to enable "nonlinear innovation" in biotechnology in the foreseeable future.

Pure resources are not enough, however. As President Kennedy noted, "New objectives and new money cannot solve these problems. They could in fact, aggravate them further—unless every scientist, every engineer, every serviceman, every technician, contractor, and civil servant gives his personal pledge that this nation will move forward."[3] In part II I discuss structural needs, such as value-based care, a continued focus on innovation, and further investment in biotechnology talent to continue to build breakthroughs. It's also important to leverage different points of view and resources, when available.

I end the book with a discussion of COVID-19 in the context of building breakthroughs, when mRNA vaccines went from idea to approval to use in near -record time. This represents a massive innovative feat.

Clinical drug development is not an easy endeavor. According to a study done by the Biotechnology Innovation Organization on clinical development success rates from 2006 to 2015, about 9.6 percent of the products, or 1 in 10, made it from initial human subject testing to FDA approval for all disease indications.[5] If you just consider oncology (cancer therapies), this number drops to 5.1 percent, or 1 in 20 products. No issue highlights the challenges of clinical drug development more than Alzheimer's, a disease affecting 5.5 million people in the United States alone, and one of the most important near-term challenges in medicine. In 1984, researchers purified a protein fragment (beta amyloid) that makes up brain plaques and described its characteristics.[6]

In subsequent years, mutations in several amyloid-related genes were linked to early-onset Alzheimer's disease, and a mouse model that overproduced beta amyloid showed increased plaque formation and memory loss that, when cleared (i.e., returned to normal), restored brain function.[7] The result of this hypothesis-driven research at the time of this writing is roughly

300 experimental drugs and billions of dollars of investment.[8] In 2021, the FDA approved Biogen/Eisai's Aduhelm (for Alzheimer's disease) under an accelerated approval pathway for reducing beta-amyloid plaque, but this decision remains controversial.[9,10]

Despite the seemingly endless complexity of medical afflictions, the trends in clinical success rates have started to improve during the past decade. A study by McKinsey and Company took the cumulative success rate from Phase I (the first step in testing a new drug treatment in humans) and broke it into smaller timeframes. It found that from 2012 through 2014, the likelihood of success was 11.6 percent.[11]

The study also noted a shift toward innovations coming from smaller companies, with partnered projects having higher success rates—an approximately 8 percent advantage over non-partnered products, particularly in the later stages. This suggests that, at an earlier point in the process, biotechnology companies have become better at identifying potential drug candidates that are likely to fail. The shift in this innovative sphere—to smaller, more focused biotechnology organizations with adequate funding, as well as related developments, including longer-term trends in the understanding of biology, the dawn of the "genomic age" of medicine, and technological advancements—has the potential to continue to revolutionize the drug development process.

I will explore how innovations in biotechnology innovation happen and discuss their creators, in conjunction with patients, entrepreneurs, and related groups of people, help shepherd these therapies from idea to reality. I hope that such stories of advancements will provide a sense of optimism, since we are indeed on the leading edge of a time when a significant change may occur in our understanding of medicine. The development of paradigm-shifting therapies that will truly impact disease outcomes for years to come.

part I

The Journey from Idea to Approval

chapter 1
Leukemia and Lymphoma

*C*ancer. The mere utterance of this word has significant meaning for everyone who hears it, producing a wide variety of reactions that run the gamut from anger to sorrow to empathy to triumph. The disease touches everybody's life. Most of us know someone who has been affected by it—a family member, a friend, a coworker, an acquaintance—or perhaps you are going through it yourself.

In their annual report on the disease, the American Cancer Society estimated that 1.9 million new cancer cases and 608,750 deaths due to the disease would occur in 2021.[1] These numbers crossed state lines and political party affiliations, with a widespread impact, ranging from 3,050 individuals in Wyoming to 187,140 in California. They also traversed age ranges. Although older people are more likely to be diagnosed with this disease, 10,500 new cancer cases were discovered among children in the 0 to 4-year-old age range in the United States in 2021. Cancer has the potential to be found in almost every part of a person's body, from the most frequent sites—in the breast (female) and prostate (male)—to rarer cancers, such as sarcomas that are located in connective tissue.

The medical and scientific communities are making significant progress against this disease, with rapid declines in death rates for the four most common cancer types in the United States— breast, prostate, lung, and colorectal—from 1990 to the present. This is attributable in part to technological breakthroughs, as well as to legislative victories, such as the National Cancer Act of 1971. From the patient's perspective, there have been significant strides in the treatment of cancer—moving from disfiguring surgeries to less invasive operations and less toxic therapeutic options. We still, however, have a long way to go.

Nonetheless, a cancer diagnosis remains a life-changing experience and comes with a whole host of emotions for diagnosed individuals, their loved ones, and their community as a whole. As Siddhartha Mukherjee writes in *The Emperor of All Maladies*, "Cancer is built into our genomes . . . and is imprinted in our society. . . . It will be a story of inventiveness, resilience, and perseverance against what one writer called the most 'relentless and insidious enemy' among human diseases."[2] Our society's saga with cancer may continue to be a series of ups and downs, but the stories of Emily Whitehead and Emily Dumler give us real hope that a new era of treatments is on the horizon.

≡ Tom Whitehead was born and raised in Phillipsburg, a town in the center of Pennsylvania with a population of 2,719, located in close proximity to Pennsylvania State University. In July 2001, Tom married his wife, Kari, on the island of Maui in Hawaii. On May 2, 2005, their first daughter, Emily, was born. Emily's initial few years of life were like those of any healthy child. She didn't sleep much her first year (which most parents of newborns can certainly relate to), and she remained healthy until after her fifth birthday. Then, on May 28, 2010, Emily woke up with leg pain, and Kari took her to see their pediatrician. Kari called Tom with the news that Emily was diagnosed with leukemia, and the family opted to start treatment at Penn State's Milton Hershey Medical Center in Hershey, Pennsylvania. The official diagnosis, confirmed on the following Tuesday, was acute lymphoblastic leukemia (ALL).

ALL is the most common cancer found in children, representing approximately 25 percent of the diagnoses in this age cohort.[3,4] In 1860, Michael Anton Biermer described the first known case of this form of childhood leukemia in Maria Speyer, the 5-year-old daughter of a carpenter in Würzburg, Germany. She exhibited severe fatigue and bruising. Biermer was called to the family's home, where he drew blood from Maria. The next afternoon, using a microscope, he defined what he saw as *exquisit Fall von Leukämie* ("an exquisite case of leukemia"). By the time Biermer returned to the family's house that evening, Maria had fallen into a coma and died, progressing from symptom to diagnosis to death in roughly three days.[2]

In 1937, Virginia senator Matthew Neely, along with other cancer-funding pioneers, such as Albert and Mary Lasker, championed a national effort to raise monies for the treatment of cancer. This led to articles published in major media sources and a general awareness campaign highlighting the lack of funding for cancer research.[5] The result of these efforts was the National Cancer Institute Act, passed unanimously by a joint session of Congress on July 23, 1937. Two weeks later, the bill was signed by President Franklin D. Roosevelt, creating the National Cancer Institute (NCI), which continues to produce groundbreaking research against the disease.

In the late 1940s, following World War II, Sidney Farber made a discovery that led to the first "temporary remissions" of the disease. He had studied biology and philosophy at the University of

Buffalo, graduating in 1923, and then trained in Germany and at Harvard Medical School. Farber eventually became the first full-time pathologist at Children's Hospital in Boston. He was intrigued by the study of aggressive tumors and took a keen interest in the development and progression of childhood leukemia.

Farber worked in the basement of the Children's Hospital. At the time, childhood leukemia was seen as a hopeless disease by most of the other physicians in the hospital, primarily due to its aggressive nature and its ability to claim lives quickly. Farber, however, noted a key finding in a journal article by physician Lucy Wills, published in *The Lancet* in 1933. She had observed that folic acid (at the time only identified as a key ingredient in Marmite, a thick commercial food paste), could have a dramatic effect if administered to pregnant women in Bombay, India, who had pernicious anemia.[6]

The direct application of folic acid in treatments for children with leukemia, however, was not that straightforward. In the initial patients Farber injected with synthetic folic acid, the disease accelerated. The rest of the pediatricians at the hospital were incensed over the results of the trial. Nonetheless, the change in the course of the disease intrigued Farber. If he could find a chemical that could block the supply of folate, it could theoretically decelerate the progression of leukemia.

At the time, Farber knew of two chemists who had folic acid blockers, Yellapragada Subbarao and Harriet Kiltie. They were able to create variants of folic acid, based on small modifications to the recipe, that were able to obstruct its action. The overall idea was to develop a molecule that would mimic folic acid and, therefore, bind to a receptor initially meant for it, a concept known as competitive inhibition.

On December 28, 1947, Farber received a package of antifolate molecules, called aminopterin, from Subbarao and Kiltie. When he injected them into a childhood leukemia patient, the response was apparent. The white blood cell count of the patient (a 2-year-old named Robert Sandler), which was increasing at an exponential rate at the time, dropped to nearly one-sixth of its peak and was within the normal range after three to four months. In January 1948, Robert was walking on his own for the first time. Two months later, his bleeding stopped, and his appetite returned.

The results of an initial study by Farber and his colleagues, published in the *New England Journal of Medicine* in 1948, described the case reports of clinical, hematologic (blood-based), and bone marrow studies in five children, selected from a total of 16 patients who were treated with aminopterin. At the time of the report, 10 of the children showed improvements lasting for three months. The remaining six patients did not respond well: four of them died, and two were diagnosed as unimproved.[7] While the results were not perfect, they were a ray of hope and were responsible for opening the era of chemotherapy for this disease.[8]

Following this initial breakthrough, in 1955 the National Cancer Institute recruited researcher Emil Freireich, who quickly befriended another man working there, Emil Frei. These two, along with Gordon Zubrod, the director of the NCI's clinical center, sought to expand on Farber's initial successes with a key idea they imported from their previous experience in the antimicrobial world. Could a combination of several drugs act in tandem to attack the cancer?

Using this hypothesis, Frei and Freireich began looking at different doses of antileukemic drugs. In 1961, they and their colleagues published a scientific journal article showing a complete remission rate of 59 percent, and a two-year survival rate of approximately 20 percent, in 39 patients when using a mixture of two drugs: mercaptopurine and methotrexate.[9] This idea of combination therapy began to catch fire in research circles, with two, three, and four types of drugs being administered together to treat the disease and bombard it from multiple angles.

Next, Donald Pinkel, at the newly opened St. Jude's Children's Research Hospital in Memphis, Tennessee, began to examine combinations of combinations. In addition to this approach, he also reasoned that injecting drug mixtures into the spinal cord, in a procedure called intrathecal administration, might be necessary, in order for them to directly reach the brain. Otherwise, several types of drugs cannot enter the brain, due to an anatomical blockade known as the blood brain barrier (BBB). This leads to relapses in patients whose tumors occur in the brain, where the cancer can evade drugs that are given intravenously. Third, Pinkel believed that such procedures should include high-dose radiation, in addition to chemical treatment, to be able to kill residual cells.[10] This approach, termed total therapy, resulted in a combination of procedures where cures were seen in approximately half of the 35 patients who were enrolled in the initial study. This stimulated similar trials that were conducted worldwide.[11–16]

≡ Today, the treatment for newly diagnosed pediatric ALL consists of a chemotherapy regimen that draws from these early breakthroughs and has three main phases: induction, consolidation, and maintenance.[12] According to the National Cancer Institute, among all children with ALL, approximately 98 percent attain remission, and approximately 85 percent of patients age 1 to 18 years with newly diagnosed ALL treated on current regimens are expected to be long-term survivors, with over 90 percent surviving for five years.[17] This highlights the impressive amount of ALL research that has yielded substantial progress against this disease. Emily Whitehead's doctors even told Tom and Kari initially that, "if you have a child with cancer, this is the one [kind of cancer] you want."

The Whiteheads were also informed that "if you follow the 26-month course of chemotherapy, she [Emily] would grow up to be a grandmother." Emily's chemotherapy treatment did not go smoothly, however. For Emily, "the first 30 days were a rough time," and, "after two rounds of chemotherapy, necrotizing fasciitis [a bacterial infection that spreads quickly] developed in both legs and she barely avoided amputiation."[18] In October 2011, when Emily went in for routine bloodwork, the doctors discovered that she was relapsing. "We were completely devastated," notes Tom. She was no longer a standard risk patient, and the chances of her survival decreased.

The next treatment protocol was to identify a donor and perform a bone marrow transplant. The Whiteheads, understandably, did not want to move forward until they received a second opinion. While they were looking for another option, Kari, who had some medical experience, since she was a research associate at Penn State, filled out what is known as an interest form, outlining Emily's situation, for the Children's Hospital of Pennsylvania at the University of Pennsylvania. Within 24 hours, Susan Rheingold, one of the leading doctors in the treatment of ALL, called Tom's cell phone to set up an appointment. "It was pretty amazing how quickly she got back to us," he remembers.

Rheingold initially confirmed what their local oncologist at Hershey Medical Center recommended—to try another round of more intense chemotherapy—but she promised that there would be more options, if necessary. In February 2012, Emily relapsed during her second course of chemotherapy, administered in preparation for a bone marrow transplant.[19] At this point, one oncologist recommended hospice care, but Tom was adamant: "That's just not how we operate." Rheingold mentioned her belief that chemo alone probably would not help Emily but said that they had a Phase I trial for an experimental drug that could be interspersed with chemo sessions. Kari researched the trial and believed it wouldn't effectively treat her daughter. Before they left the hospital, Rheingold said one more thing that would alter the course of Emily's story: "You turned down this trial and chemo,

[but] you're going to have to pick something, and I just want to tell you there's this upcoming T cell trial that's two to three months away from FDA approval, and we think it could work."

The Whiteheads returned to Hershey Medical Center and decided to give Emily another round of chemo. This knocked her cancer back briefly and bought them about three more weeks, until the head of the oncology team, John Neely, said to Tom, "We don't have any more weapons to fight this cancer." Out of options, Tom and Kari called Rheingold, who serendipitously had just received an email stating that the FDA had given the Children's Hospital of Philadelphia permission to treat their first patient with T cells. On March 1, 2012, Emily was transferred to the Children's Hospital of Philadelphia and met Stephen Grupp. What came next would alter the course of history for the treatment of pediatric ALL.

≡ It was a typical summer day on August 8, 2013, when Emily Dumler experienced some stomach pain: "It didn't feel great, but it didn't feel horrible either." Emily, the mother of three young children, was at a friend's house, with the kids playing outside, so she didn't think much of it. When Emily arrived back home, she found a substantial amount of blood in her stool. Alarmed, Emily called her primary care physician and headed to an urgent care center. The medical staff ran some initial blood tests, which showed very low platelet counts, so much so that the doctor believed the technician may have made an error, so he ordered a retest. When the results confirmed that her platelet count was in the 1,000 range, the lowest the physician had ever seen, Emily sensed that something was wrong, although she commented, "At this point I don't even know what platelets are, so this is all new to me."

Emily Dumler hails from a big Kansas family. Her mother is one of 11 kids, and Emily has 26 cousins. Up until this point, none of her family members had had cancer or any serious illness: "I didn't really have any experience, and I was completely clueless about what it was, really." The doctors at the urgent care center were not sure what was causing her low platelet count, either, so they made a preliminary diagnosis of idiopathic thrombocytopenic purpura, or ITP, a bleeding disorder where the immune system destroys the body's platelets, which are needed for blood clotting. To her, it almost felt like a diagnosis by exclusion. This inconclusive finding led from what Emily thought would be a quick trip to an urgent care center for a stomach bug to admittance to the hospital for 43 days: "It was scary more than anything. I was sad and lonely with the kids [left] at home. My husband had to work and take care of the kids, but friends and family were volunteering anywhere they could."

At the hospital, she underwent several therapies to increase her platelet count, such as steroids, a splenectomy, and intravenous immunoglobulin therapy, which is used for patients with ITP. Her entire body was bruised from the four blood draws per day and the various treatments she received. Put on a liquid diet to receive additional calories, she still lost 8 to 10 pounds, and the community hospital staff remained stumped by her lack of response. She was then transferred to the University of Kansas Medical Center, where medical personnel performed her first CT and PET scans. These found signs of diffuse large B-cell lymphoma, or DLBCL. According to the Lymphoma Research Foundation, DLBCL is an aggressive (fast-growing) form of cancer that can arise either in the lymph nodes or outside the lymphatic system. An initial painless, rapid swelling in the neck or other areas is then followed by other symptoms, such as fever, unexplained weight loss, and fatigue.

Thomas Hodgkin was born to a Quaker family in Pentonville, St. James Parish, Middlesex, in the United Kingdom, and received his medical training at St. Thomas's and Guy's Medical School. In 1832, Hodgkin published an article in which he described several cases he deemed "probably familiar to many practical morbid anatomists . . . and have not (as far as I am aware) been made the subject of special attention."[20] In 1865, almost 30 years after this initial paper, Samuel Wilks, a British physician, named the disease for the author. It is now known as Hodgkin's lymphoma. Subsequently, the medical community grouped other lymph node enlargements that weren't categorized as Hodgkin's lymphoma into a second, catchall category: non-Hodgkin's lymphoma, or NHL. This duality remained until the late 1950s, when the multiple forms of NHL were categorized into what was termed the Rappaport classification.[21]

≡ On December 2, 1943, the Germans bombed an Allied port in Bari, on the coast of Italy, sinking 17 ships and killing more than 1,000 American and British servicemen, as well as hundreds of civilians. The most seriously hit ship in the attack, the SS *John Harvey*, was carrying a secret cargo of 2,000 mustard gas bombs, to potentially be used in retaliation if Hitler resorted to gas warfare.[22] This tragedy led to a unique observation: both the bone marrow and the lymph nodes of the men exposed to mustard gas were severely depleted.

Milton Winternitz, dean of the Yale School of Medicine, obtained a contract from the US Office of Scientific Research and Development, due to his previous work on sulfur mustards during World War I, and directed two pharmacologists at Yale, Alfred Gilman and Louis Goodman, to examine the potential therapeutic effects of mustard gases. The researchers found significant tumor regressions in mouse experiments and convinced their colleague, Gustaf Lindskog, a thoracic surgeon, to administer nitrogen mustard to a patient with NHL and severe airway obstruction. The impressive results were published in 1946, three years after the studies were performed, due to the secrecy associated with this wartime gas program.[23–25]

The results of the study set off a burst of research in NHL. The remissions seen with nitrogen mustard turned out to be brief and incomplete, however, similar to Farber's initial folic acid study. Vincent DeVita came to the NCI in 1963 and immediately began to collaborate with colleagues like Zubrod, Frei, and Freireich. They developed a protocol known as MOMP—which included nitrogen mustard, vincristine (Oncovin), methotrexate, and prednisone, and combination regimens with nitrogen mustard began to enter clinical trials in the treatment of Hodgkin's lymphoma and NHL.

MOMP eventually was revised into an improved protocol by replacing methotrexate with a more powerful drug, called procarbazine, for a regimen known as MOPP, and, subsequently, became a regimen known as C-MOPP, which replaced nitrogen mustard with a drug called cyclophosphamide. The use of chemotherapy was a game changer in the treatment of lymphomas. A field that had previously been derided as crazy and potentially dangerous became not just reputable, but an accepted new avenue of treatment.[26] Further work in characterizing the pathology of NHL led to descriptions of subsets of the disease, called diffuse histiocytic lymphoma (now known as DLBCL), which accounts for approximately 30–40 percent of new cases.[27]

DeVita and his colleagues published the results of a 1975 study, showing that showed 11 of 27 patients treated with C-MOPP achieved complete remission of their cancerous tumors, with 10 of them free of all evidence for 26 to 105 months from the end of treatment, a remarkable result for the time.[28] As noted in a study published in the *New England Journal of Medicine*, "The development of curative combination chemotherapy for patients with advanced stages of aggressive non-Hodgkin's lymphoma has been one of the major successes of cancer therapy."[29]

In this stream of combination therapy research, which extended for several decades (and continues to be tinkered with even today, as newer and safer alternatives are developed), a chemotherapy regimen using a combination of four drugs known as CHOP—cyclophosphamide, doxorubicin (hydroxydaunomycin), vincristine (Oncovin), and prednisolone—became the standard of care for the majority of patients with NHL in the later part of the past century, but there are still a subset of patients who do not respond to this therapy.

≡ To confirm Emily Dumler's diagnosis, following the finding of DLBCL in her scans, her physicians needed to get a biopsy tissue sample and increase her platelet counts via chemotherapy. Around day 40 in the hospital, the doctors performed a colonoscopy for the biopsy, as the tumor was in a part of her intestine known as the ileum. During the procedure, Emily had to have four blood transfusions to maintain her platelet count at an acceptable level. The biopsy confirmed the presence of DLBCL, and her doctors labeled it as stage 3, or locally advanced cancer. "Honestly, I was relieved to finally have a diagnosis," Emily recalls, and she was discharged the following day.

Her subsequent treatment plan began with six rounds of chemotherapy, with a regimen known as R-CHOP. The *R* stands for a drug known as rituximab, which targets a receptor, known as CD20, on the surface of B cells and is used in combination with CHOP. In a landmark study, previously untreated patients with DLBCL showed a complete response (the absence of all detectable cancer after the treatment is finished) of 76 percent with R-CHOP versus 63 percent with CHOP, along with a significantly longer duration of their remissions and overall survival times. In other words, over two-thirds of the patients treated with R-CHOP would be in remission for two years or more.[30] The side effects of this therapy are those occurring in most cancer treatments: hair loss, exhaustion, and nausea.

The setting within an infusion center can vary from hospital to hospital. The center Emily Dumler went to had four long rows of reclining chairs, where patients sat and received their therapies via intravenous infusion. As she has commented, "When you're getting treatment, you feel good because you're actually doing something. It's the waiting that's the hard part, because you aren't doing anything." At the halfway point of her therapy, the scans showed that her cancer was already in remission. By the end of February 2014, Emily believed she was cancer free.

Nonetheless, on another lazy summer day, roughly one year after she had initially found out she had cancer, Emily went to her doctor for a follow-up colonoscopy and heard the news that the cancer was still there. She then had an autologous stem cell transplant, where cells are extracted from the patient's bone marrow and are reinfused following a high-dose chemotherapy regimen. After her cancer had progressed still further, another option was an allogeneic transplant, where a healthy donor's cells are infused into the patient. This procedure, however, comes with additional risks, such as the donor cells viewing the patient's healthy cells as foreign and attacking them—a condition called graft-versus-host disease. As Emily recalls, "Now that I was more familiar with the research, I was terrified, since there were so many more risks involved with the allogeneic transplant." While waiting for a donor match, she went to the M. D. Anderson Cancer Center in Houston, Texas, for another opinion and learned about a different type of autologous stem cell transplant, using the immune system's T cells. This treatment would require her to move to Houston for three months, and, in the end, Emily and her family came to the conclusion that the benefits outweighed the risks.

In December 2014, Emily Dumler went to Houston to receive her therapies and spent a large portion of the time there by herself, with different caregivers coming both to visit her and to stay at home with her kids. As she notes, "We piecemealed it." The treatment was no walk in the park. Mouth sores limited her ability to eat or swallow. She lost 20 pounds and was now a 5'4" woman weighing around 88 pounds. The doctors would try to keep her active by getting her to walk, but there were several days where she was in too much pain or too tired to do so. By the end of February 2015, she completed her therapy at the M. D. Anderson Center and went back to Kansas City, unsure of what would come next.

≡ Emily Dumler's story, like Emily Whitehead's, would be transformed by an investigational T cell therapy trial that was the result of several years of medical research, leading to a breakthrough. Their stories align with Siddhartha Mukherjee's description of the ongoing treatment of cancer as one of "inventiveness, resilience, and perseverance,"[2] and they provide hope that we are developing new tools to fight the disease.

chapter 2
Chimeric Antigen Receptor (CAR)-T Cell Therapy

I n 2005, Steve Jobs gave a commencement speech at Stanford University that related three stories from his experience. In reflecting on the purpose of them in the trajectory of his life, he opined, "You can't connect the dots looking forward; you can only connect them looking backwards. So you have to trust that the dots will somehow connect in your future. You have to trust in something—your gut, destiny, life, karma, whatever."[1] When Capt. Carl June, MD, now a director at the Abramson Cancer Center at the University of Pennsylvania, has looked back on a series of circumstances from his life that led to this book's first example of a breakthrough in medicine, he humbly and unbelievably shakes his head in agreement with Jobs.

Carl has a strong build, standing roughly six feet tall, with the broad shoulders befitting a military officer. He was born in 1953 in Golden, Colorado, where his father studied at the Colorado School of Mines. After a stint at Aberdeen Proving Grounds in Maryland during his father's Korean War army service, the family landed in Emeryville, California, where his father worked as a chemical engineer at Shell Development, a research organization operated by Shell Oil.

At a very young age, Carl took to biology, conducting experiments at home. In elementary school, he and a friend purchased some rats, anesthetized them with carbon tetrachloride—a cleaning fluid widely used in the 1960s, before its effects on human health and the environment were discovered, leading to the Consumer Product Safety Commission banning its use in consumer products in the United States in the 1970s[2]—made a midline incision, and then sutured the cuts closed. While Carl claims that that it was technically a successful experiment, he is quick to provide the caveat (with a dry chuckle) that his younger self did not realize the rats would chew the sutures a few days later. He notes, "I'm not sure my mom and dad ever found out we did that."

Other experiments were not as easily hidden. Another homegrown attempt from a curious young Carl involved starting his father's barbeque grill, taking his mother's vacuum cleaner, and reversing the flow, to try to make hot air balloons: "That didn't work out too well, since the motor on the vacuum cleaner was melted by the barbeque. . . . Mom and dad certainly found out about that one and weren't too happy, to say the least." As Carl was naturally curious and inquisitive, he excelled in primary and secondary school, with Gary Pasi, his eighth-grade biology teacher, helping to nurture his initial interest. He was the valedictorian of his graduating class of 400 students at College Park High School, which "was an amazingly flexible school that let me take college courses." This occasion was the first of his now thousands of public speaking events, but "I still remember how I was scared to death to give that speech."

In 1971, a teenaged Carl received an acceptance letter from Stanford University and was prepared to follow in his father's and brother's footsteps, becoming an engineer. Instead, Jobs's "gut, destiny, life, karma, whatever" intervened. Carl's draft lottery number for the Vietnam War was 50, and, as he explains, "that year, about the first 150 went, and at [number] 50, I was right up there." Instead of waiting to be drafted, he instead chose to enroll in the US Naval Academy. He thought this would allow him to continue his pursuit of engineering while fulfilling his military obligation. He even spent a summer on a nuclear submarine.

He then decided to attend medical school, with the costs entirely paid for by the Navy, in exchange for extended military service. Carl was accepted at all three institutions he applied to, including Harvard. He notes, however, "I was not allowed to go there, even though it was my first choice, because the ROTC [Reserve Officers' Training Corps] was off campus at the time, due to war protests." In the meantime, his parents moved from the San Francisco Bay area to Houston, so Carl went to Baylor College of Medicine. "I actually finished in three years, thinking I could get out of a year of obligation, but no deal." When he graduated, he owed 12 years of service to the Navy, as part of the agreement for funding his educational pursuits.

During this time, another chance occurrence shaped Carl's career trajectory. The potential use of nuclear weapons in the war meant that doctors needed to understand radiation toxicity. This required further knowledge about bone marrow transplants, the only effective treatment for radiation poisoning. In another sequence of unplanned events, Carl, who was keen on pursuing research interests at that time, and three other physicians were sent to the Fred Hutchinson Cancer Research Center in Seattle to learn about this procedure. Bone marrow is a spongy tissue that exists inside certain bones. It contains stem cells, which have the ability to develop into red blood cells (that carry oxygen), platelets (that help with blood clotting), or white blood cells (that make up a portion of your immune system).

Bone marrow transplants can use either your own cells, in a

process known as autologous transplantation, or cells from a healthy matched donor, in a process known as allogeneic transplantation. One category of white blood cells is known as T cells, or T lymphocytes. These play a key role in recognizing foreign substances in a person's body and helping to attack them with what is known as a T cell receptor (or TCR). Carl's key takeaway from his experience in Seattle was that he "learned quickly that T cells had the potential to kill you more rapidly than leukemia could."

Carl began his training at the Fred Hutchinson Center in 1983 and finished in mid-1986. His experiences there were invaluable and would contribute to his interest in using the body's immune system to fight diseases. He took these lessons to Bethesda, Maryland, in 1987, where, at the age of 31, he started his own laboratory at the Naval Medical Research Institute. The lab was paid for the National Institutes of Health. Carl initially focused on using T cells to treat HIV. NIH funding at this juncture in his career was key, because Carl "didn't have to worry about writing long grant proposals and could just focus on doing the research." Carl, along with his postdoctoral associate, Bruce Levine, published several important papers on growing T cells and helped discover CD28, a biological pathway that allowed T cells to attack other cells. This would prove to be valuable in using T cells to treat cancer.[3,4]

During this period, Zelig Eshhar, from the Weizmann Institute of Science in Rehovot, Israel, began presenting intriguing data on the ability to reengineer TCRs with antibody therapies, positing a potential new approach to treat cancer. This was an important step for the field, because with this approach, the immune system would be able to overcome its initial inability to recognize cancer cells. In addition to this work, several key research groups in the United States—including Carl June's at the University of Pennsylvania, Steve Rosenberg's at the National Cancer Institute, Michael Jensen's at the City of Hope cancer research center, and Michel Sadelain's at Memorial Sloan Kettering Cancer Center in

New York City—began to make discoveries that allowed T cells to be reengineered to attack cancer cells. This led to the emergence of CAR-T [Chimeric Antigen Receptor-T cell] therapy, the first example of a breakthrough in medicine that I will explore.

≡ A CAR is a special receptor that allows a T cell to target cancerous tumor cells in a focused manner. The first therapeutic CAR-Ts were created by collecting T cells from a patient via a blood withdrawal; genetically reengineering the cell to allow it to produce a CAR protein that targets the cancer; multiplying these genetically modified T cells; and then re-infusing them into the patient. CARs were initially made at the University of California at San Francisco for basic scientific purposes.[5] In 1991, Carl June and his colleagues retargeted T cells using that technology,[6] and the resulting product was licensed to a biotechnology company called Cell Genesys, in order to treat HIV. (The first CAR-T trial was actually conducted in HIV patients.)

Cell Genesys conducted three clinical trials that showed evidence of benefits from targeted T cells in HIV, but newer and easier-to-administer therapies for the disease, called proteasome inhibitors, were introduced in 1997. That development, along with a lack of funding (due to a high profile death occurring in a clinical trial) forced Cell Genesys to go belly up.

At this turn of events, Carl June assumed sponsorship of the study, due to a National Institutes of Health requirement that patients in gene therapy trials had to be followed for 15 years after treatment (a rule that still exists today). When he examined cells from all 40 patients that were involved in the studies, with an initial intent of putting the CAR-T therapy to rest, Carl and his team found that the modified T cells had a therapeutic duration of more than 17 years. Despite a dearth of funding, he and the other CAR-T pioneers continued to push forward. This issue became particularly personal when Carl's wife Cynthia was diagnosed with ovarian cancer in 1996 and passed away in 2001: "After what happened to my wife, I started working on that [CAR technology to cure cancer] full time."[7]

≡ When Tom, Kari, and Emily Whitehead met Stephen Grupp at the Children's Hospital of Philadelphia, they didn't know what to expect. As Tom explains it, "He was a straight-shooter; he doesn't sugarcoat it in any way. He was a phenomenal person in addition to a great doctor, and we felt confident in him the first time we spoke." Grupp warned the Whiteheads, "I can't tell you for sure this will work for Emily's cancer." As of 2010, several adult patients with chronic lymphocytic leukemia had received CAR-T therapy, with robust antileukemic effects.[8,9] Instead, Emily, who was a child suffering from refractory and relapsed acute lymphoblastic leukemia (ALL), was to be the first pediatric patient. In general, there are differences in treating children, compared with adults, that can be attributed to body size, various stages of growth, and so forth. These can make the direct translation of a drug's efficacy (i.e., it's power to produce a desired effect) from one age bracket to the other difficult. Nonetheless, at this point, the Whiteheads had exhausted all other options to treat Emily's cancer.

On April 17, 2012, Emily Whitehead became the first pediatric patient treated with CAR-T therapy. Thus Carl June and Stephen Grupp split the dose of T cells over three days—10 percent on day 1, 30 percent on day 2, and 60 percent on day 3—while monitoring safety measures and Emily's tolerance of the product. "It was scary, but we had a lot of hope, and we needed to think outside the box," Tom remembers. After the full dose was given, Emily became critically ill. She was admitted to the pediatric intensive care unit with multiorgan failure and a 106° fever. This side effect, known as cytokine release syndrome, or CRS, can occur in varying degrees of severity after a large influx of an immunotherapy treatment (such as T cells) is administered. As the

Whiteheads note, "Nothing prepared us for the CRS. It was the worst thing we'd ever seen."

The processes developed to mitigate this side effect included a split dosage (which was already included in the clinical trial protocol); steroid treatment; or treatment with another drug, one that's used for arthritis, which blocks a protein called tumor necrosis factor, or TNF. CRS was also seen in the first adult patient receiving modified CAR-T cells in 2010, 72-year-old Bill Ludwig, but he recovered from the side effect without additional therapy. To help relieve some of the problems with Emily, the doctors gave her a high dose of steroids, but nothing happened. They then tried the anti-TNF drug, but that didn't work, either. At this point, the attending doctors were out of treatment options and were very worried that Emily could die. The Pediatric Intensive Care Unit staff placed Emily in a medically induced coma, and Grupp and his team began looking for options. As Tom recalls, "Kari and I would talk in her ear and play her favorite songs, anything we could do to connect with her."

During this time, Michael Kalos was performing laboratory tests of proteins in Emily's blood and had sent the workups to Carl June, who was traveling from Seattle to Houston to give presentations to fellow colleagues on the progress to date of CAR-T therapy. Emily's fever had spiked on Friday, after initially being dosed with the cells on Tuesday. According to Carl, "I had drafted an email to the chancellor [of the University of Pennsylvania] on Saturday, and we honestly believed that she was going to die on Sunday," reflecting that "when the first pediatric patient passes away in a clinical trial, it is very difficult to have faith in trying it [on] another patient for a long time." So how did Emily survive and help pave the way for this breakthrough?

The answer lies in perhaps the most significant alignment of dots in this amazing story. On the plane from Seattle to Houston, Carl noticed an elevation of two key proteins in Kalos's tests: one for a protein known as interferon-gamma, and the other for a protein called interleukin-6, or IL-6 for short. The increase in IL-6 was what particularly caught his eye, as this rise could be seen over the three days of Emily's split dosages. More importantly, Carl's daughter, who is now almost in her 30s, had juvenile rheumatoid arthritis.

In 2009, Carl was president of the Clinical Immunological Society, where he presented an award to Tadamitsu Kishmoto, a Japanese researcher who developed the drug tocilizumab, targeting IL-6. This drug was subsequently licensed to the health care company Roche, and in 2010 it was approved for the treatment of rheumatoid arthritis. How many other oncologists would have had this in-depth knowledge about a drug being developed for rheumatoid arthritis? "Not many, if any at all," Carl guesses. Again, according to the quote from Steve Jobs, "you can't connect the dots looking forward; you can only connect them looking backwards."

As a result of this connection, Carl was able to secure some of the drug. Because Emily was a pediatric patient, her parents had to consent to the off label use of tocilizumab—that is, employing the drug to treat a condition for which it had not been officially approved. Grupp used this therapy with Emily, and within hours of its administration, she woke up from her coma with no fever. Coincidentally it was also Emily's seventh birthday—May 2, 2012. As Tom now says proudly, "She may grow close to 6 feet tall." The case study was subsequently published in the *New England Journal of Medicine* in 2013, noting the remarkable result[10]

"It was miraculous," Carl says. Even though he's probably retold this story hundreds of times, he notes, "It doesn't get any less miraculous every time I tell it." He also agrees wholeheartedly with Steve Jobs's quote: "I couldn't have imagined that all the random events in my life would have connected to lead me here." When Emily was recovering, Tom and Kari asked the staff if they could tour the lab where this therapy was created. When they met Carl, emotions ran high, particularly given the age of the latter's young daughter. Tom recalls, "Carl's first words to us were, 'Sorry she got so sick.'"

Since her remission, Emily's story spread like wildfire in research circles and major media outlets. She and her parents have attended Stand Up to Cancer events, as well as being featured in newspapers, magazines, and Ken Burns's *Emperor of All Maladies* documentary. "I never thought I'd need a media lawyer," Tom Whitehead quips, "but now all we want to do is tell Emily's story to help as many patients with cancer as possible receive treatment." Emily, her parents, and the staff at Children's Hospital, including Carl June and Stephen Grupp, have helped write the next chapter in therapy for pediatric acute lymphoblastic leukemia. Fortunately, CAR-Ts are not a "one-trick pony," and the Whiteheads' focus on telling their story has helped many other patients seeking treatment, including Emily Dumler.

☰ On a rainy spring day in April 2015, almost two months following Emily Dumler's autologous transplant at the M. D. Anderson Cancer Center, she sat in her living room in Kansas City. She had a gut feeling that something was wrong. Although she was slowly regaining weight from her previous procedure, when she went in for a checkup, it revealed what she already felt she knew—her transplant was unsuccessful. "I was devastated," she comments when recalling the news. Her doctors had given her six months to live, with her only treatment option being an allogeneic stem cell transplant, using cells from a donor, which carries several risks. The prognosis was grim. The transplant had only a 10 percent chance of being successful, and even then, the side effects of this therapy were unknown. As Emily recalls, "I questioned a lot of things in this time, including whether or not it was worth it to buy clothes for the upcoming winter or if it would be a waste of money." In the end, though, both for herself and for her family, she knew she had to hold it together.

When Emily Dumler went to the University of Kansas Medical Center, her physician noted that there was a clinical trial for CAR-T cells being used in patients with diffuse large B-cell lymphoma, which was her diagnosis. When Emily looks back on this moment, she can't help but wonder, "If I had the original allogeneic transplant, it could've worked, but who knows what side effects I would be dealing with. More importantly, if I [had] had it, I wouldn't have been able to enroll in the study." She was familiar with Emily Whitehead's story from the HBO series *VICE*, which had chronicled the latter's journey in late February 2015, when she was finishing what would be her last autologous stem cell treatment. Emily Dunbar's doctor at the University of Kansas Medical Center called the M. D. Anderson Center and was told that they had one spot available in the clinical trial for DLBCL, which was beginning the following week.

≡ Kite Pharma sponsored the clinical trial Emily Dumler was enrolled in. The company was founded in 2009 by Arie Belldegrun. He went to medical school in Israel, finished his postgraduate studies at the Weizmann Institute of Science, and completed his residency at Brigham and Women's Hospital in Cambridge, Massachusetts. In 1985 he started a research fellowship with Steve Rosenberg at the National Cancer Institute. Immunotherapy was in its infancy then, and Rosenberg was a pioneer. As he recalls, "There was something special about Arie. He was extremely smart, hard working, and driven by a passion to develop treatments for patients. We saw in each other kindred spirits and became good friends."

In *Zero to One: Notes on Startups*, by Peter Thiel and Blake Masters, they address the contentious question of whether great achievements come from luck or from skill. While many successful people are quick to claim luck—Warren Buffet considers himself a "member of the lucky sperm club" as well as a winner of the "ovarian lottery," and Bill Gates says he "was lucky to be born with certain skills"—the authors note that "the phenomenon of serial entrepreneurship would seem to call into question our tendency to explain success as the product of chance. If success were mostly a matter of luck, these kinds of serial entrepreneurs probably wouldn't exist."[11] Belldegrun fits the criteria of a flourishing serial entrepreneur in biotechnology, and he has taken significant steps to advance cancer therapies. As noted in a *New York Times* article written about Kite Pharma, "Dr. Belldegrun . . . has commercial flair. [He] seems as comfortable on Wall Street or in high society as in the operating room."[12]

In 1988, Belldegrun moved to the University of California, Los Angeles and cofounded a biotech company, Agensys. Astellas Pharma acquired it in 2007 for $537 million. He was then involved in the formation of Cougar Biotechnology in 2009, which developed the blockbuster late-stage prostate cancer drug now known as Zytiga. Cougar was later sold to Johnson & Johnson for $970 million. The name "Kite" originated as a result of the Johnson & Johnson / Cougar transaction. When putting together deals, code names are often assigned to cloak the true identity of the participating firms. Johnson & Johnson used the name Kite for the transaction, and when the deal was completed, Belldegrun trademarked the name for his new company.

In 2012 and 2013, Kite entered into a cooperative research and development agreement (CRADA) with the National Cancer Institute to undertake a study of anti-CD19 CAR-T therapy in humans, and the company also licensed intellectual property from Zelig Eshhar. As Rosenberg recalls, "An indication of his brilliant insight is that Arie realized it [the promise of cell therapies] long before most people." At this time, Kite was a startup in every sense of the word. The first building (on 2225 Colorado Avenue in Santa Monica, California) was located next to the Santa Monica Department of Motor Vehicles and had faulty air conditioning and plumbing.

In May 2013, the company completed a $35 million Series A preferred stock financing. (Series A financing represents the initial venture capital funding for a startup). This stage built on the initial $15 million raised in March 2011. Kite then hired its chief financial officer, Cynthia ("Cindy") Butitta, in late 2013. Up until this point, Belldegrun had served as the executive chairman of the board, but in March 2014, Kite's board of directors and, specifically, board member David Bonderman, said that Belldegrun was the only one who could be the chief executive officer (CEO) of the company. With Belldegrun officially at the helm, Kite completed its initial public offering on June 20, 2014. By the close of the stock market on day 1 of the public offering, its worth was up by roughly 54 percent, with a valuation close to $1 billion.

In August 2014, the National Cancer Institute published results of their Phase I/IIa clinical trial of aggressive non-Hodgkin's lymphoma (NHL) patients receiving anti-CD19 CAR-T therapy. Of the 13 participants who were evaluated, 12 of them either had complete remissions (8 patients) or partial remissions (4 patients), for a 92 percent objective (or overall) response rate—that is, the percentage of patients whose tumor size was reduced over a specified time period. The astonishing results supported Kite's plan to file an investigational new drug (IND) application to initiate a Phase I/II study with the product, called KTE-C19, for the treatment of patients with refractory (treatment-resistant) aggressive NHL.

≡ Emily Dumler's T cells were collected at the end of May and sent to California to be engineered at Kite. She received her T cell therapy on July 13, 2015, as the third participant in Kite's Phase I/II study. After therapy, she immediately developed a 39.5°C

(103.1 °F) fever, which eventually developed into CRS. Like Emily Whitehead, Emily Dumler received tocilizumab and promptly responded to the treatment. When the latter was in the hospital, the doctors completed several checks daily on her neurological functions. On day 5 after receiving therapy, she was asked to jot down where she was from. Emily attempted to write "Shawnee [Kansas] is beautiful," but she could not remember how to spell the word "beautiful." She tried to think of a different term but could not do that, either. As Emily later recalls, "What was the scariest thing about the whole post-treatment process was not being able to remember my son's name. His name is Hudson, but I called him 'Spanish.'"

Fortunately, a second dose of tocilizumab seemed to do the trick and resolved Emily Dumler's neurotoxicity issues. Nine days after she received CAR-T therapy, she was discharged from the hospital; on day 30 she was declared in complete remission. Her case study was the third confirmed case of a DLBCL remission, and it was published as part of a larger review in the journal *Nature Reviews Clinical Oncology*: "[This case study] does not illustrate the most severe toxicities observed after CAR-T therapy, although it does reflect the most common observed clinical scenario."[13]

Emily Dumler, however, does not view her situation as "common" at all. Further, she notes that as an early participant in a clinical trial, "I would've thought that I would be terrified and hopeless, but in actuality, I have to say that I felt the opposite. I felt positive and hopeful." Emily is quick to suggest that seeing Emily Whitehead's miraculous and remarkable story kept her thinking "that could be me" during her treatment for DLBCL. Due to the courage, strength, and resolve shown by them, the doctors and scientists associated with the development of this therapy, and the entrepreneurs who saw its potential, CAR-Ts are able to treat many more patients with these types of leukemia and lymphoma. And this breakthrough for the treatment of cancer may only be the beginning.

≡ Michael Jensen went to medical school at the University of Pennsylvania, specializing in pediatrics. He then received a fellowship at the University of Washington Medical School and the Fred Hutchinson Cancer Center (also referred to as "The Hutch") in Seattle. As Jensen notes, "My grandfather was involved in the development of the vaccine for diphtheria and he served as my guiding light for a career in science." During his early education, Jensen was able to work with Phillip Greenberg at The Hutch: "I would say that he and Steve Rosenberg were pioneers in immuno-oncology." Jensen was also impressed by Zelig Eshhar's work. In 1997, when Jensen became an assistant professor at the City of Hope, a cancer-focused treatment hospital northeast of Los Angeles, he concentrated on the development of CAR-T cells to treat cancer. In 2007, Jensen, along with Stan Riddell from The Hutch, started a company called ZetaRx to further develop their academic discoveries.

Later they, together with Michel Sadelain, Isabelle Rivière, and Renier Brentjens from the Memorial Sloan Kettering Cancer Center, became scientific cofounders of Juno Therapeutics (one of the initial names for the company was FC Therapeutics, with the "FC" standing for "F*** Cancer"), which acquired ZetaRx. As their first project, Juno Therapeutics was focused on treating DL-BCL with CAR-T cells, similar to what Kite Pharma did. To make the jump from academic endeavor to potential commercial product, they needed a catalyst. As Jensen notes, "For Juno, Bob Nelsen was really the spark that activated the leadership of The Hutch. When he saw the data [Bob sat on the board of the Fred Hutchinson Cancer Center at the time], he said that it was too good, you have to start a company."

Bob Nelsen, a managing partner at ARCH Venture Partners, is known for taking big, bold risks in biotechnology. He has invested in companies that range from the now multibillion-dollar gene sequencer firm Illumina, to the infectious disease–focused biotechnology company Vir Biotechnology, to the biopharmaceutical manufacturing and technology enterprise Resilience. Bob has helped create, source, finance, and develop more than 150 companies, with over 30 having reached billion-dollar valuations, landing him at number 48 on *Forbes* magazine's 2021 Midas List for world's top venture capital investors.[14]

Nelsen grew up in Walla Walla, Washington, picking strawberries, and initially thought anybody he worked with had to have that farming mentality. Nelsen recently said to a group of University of California, San Francisco students, "I think my strongest attribute was persistence. When I wanted to get into venture capital, I called Brooke Byers [a prominent venture capitalist for Kleiner Perkins Caufield & Byers] 35 times until he finally called me back."

He clearly had a strong interest in public markets at an early age, trading stocks as an 11-year-old and clerking at the Chicago Board Options Exchange in his late teens. Nelsen stayed closer to home for his undergraduate degree, majoring in biology and economics at the University of Puget Sound, and received his MBA from the University of Chicago.[15] When he joined ARCH Venture Partners, its purpose was to commercialize academic intellectual property. In part this arose after a University of Chicago professor who failed to patent a method for making a scalable, recombinant erythropoietin, or EPO, a drug that is commonly known for its use in blood doping in the Tour de France. It also came about because there was a multibillion-dollar commercial market for biotechnology companies.

In 1992, ARCH split from the University of Chicago and became a separate investment entity. Nelsen saw CAR-T therapy as a way "to fundamentally transform cancer therapy." Given his track record, once he is focused on a big problem, he will attempt to solve it. As Jensen notes, "Bob was critical to the formation of the company. He had a vision of how to put this [Juno Therapeutics] together and do it big and fast. He was able to deliver on it."

Organizational psychology research has advocated the potential benefits of an "outsider advantage": the more information that specialists create, the greater the opportunity for generalists to draw new conclusions from it.[16] Taking cellular therapies from idea to approval required a mixture of different specialties, along with some serendipity and luck. The idea itself involved prior knowledge, generated from the field of bone marrow transplants; the concept of using one's own cells as a form of treatment; and immunology, employing T cells to attack cancer. Serendipity came from a doctor who happened to have a child with juvenile rheumatoid arthritis.

The CAR-T landscape also highlights the fragile nature of competition and collaboration that is unique to both the development of medicines and an understanding of biology. Following early successes, such as those seen with Emily Whitehead and Emily Dumler, the race to develop commercial CAR-T therapies was on. In this first example of a breakthrough, the University of Pennsylvania / Novartis, Kite Pharma, and Juno Therapeutics were initially looking to treat ALL and DLBCL patients with cellular therapies. These biotech companies were considered to be the leaders in the field, competing to advance CAR-T treatments and eying the potential to commercialize them.

chapter 3
Spinal Muscular Atrophy

The birth of a first child is a both an exciting and a terrifying experience. It's a journey into the unknown: Will we be good parents? Will our lives truly change forever? On November 20, 2011, Derwin Almeida and his girlfriend Nicole married and moved into a home in Miami, Florida. Derwin found out he was going to be an uncle when his sister learned she was pregnant. During her pregnancy, she had been told that she was a carrier for a genetic disease called spinal muscular atrophy (SMA). She immediately informed Nicole that Derwin was probably a carrier as well and should get tested. "When my sister told us that she was a carrier, it was really an afterthought at the time, we didn't know what it [SMA] was, and we weren't even sure at the time if and when we were going to have kids," Derwin recalls. "We don't have any family history of genetic disease in our family, either."

In the fall of 2014, Nicole went to see her doctor for her annual visit. She mentioned that they were going to start trying to have a child and asked about being tested for SMA. As Nicole recalls,

"She [my doctor] told me that the test was not covered by our insurance and that it would be about $2,500. I told her I would talk to my husband and then make the appointment. I spoke to my husband and we agreed to do the genetic testing, but by the time my appointment came around I was already pregnant."

Nicole, a paralegal, made it a point to research everything: "Whenever people in the family need something looked up, they come to me." When she had her next checkup, on December 12, she and Derwin decided to be tested for SMA: "I found out I was a carrier and we went in the next day and had him tested. The tests confirmed he was a carrier, and at the time I was already four months pregnant, so I was referred to a high-risk doctor for an amniocentesis." Amniocentesis is a procedure that samples the amniotic fluid, using a needle that is inserted into the uterus. It screens for developmental abnormalities and is performed approximately 200,000 times per year. Nonetheless, it poses potential risks, such as miscarriage.[1]

On March 3, 2015, Nicole and Derwin received a call from their doctor asking them to come in to discuss the test results. As Derwin notes, "We were nervous about hearing the result when they called us in, but thought, 'Let's just be positive.'" When they arrived for their appointment, the doctor confirmed their fears. Nicole remembers hearing, "Your child has SMA type 1; he's probably going to die before his first birthday. Here's an abortion paper, or you can have him and enjoy that time with him." At that point, she recalls, "We were devastated. We had no idea what the disease was, and the doctors in Miami had little information, because it is a rare disease."

☰ SMA affects roughly 1 in 11,000 babies and is the number one genetic cause of death for infants. About 1 in every 50 Americans is a genetic carrier. SMA is a disease that degrades the body's physical strength by affecting the motor nerve cells in the spinal cord, taking away the ability to walk, eat, or breathe.[2] The most severe form of the disease, referred to as SMA type 1, is also called Werdnig-Hoffman disease, based on findings in 1891 from an Austrian neurologist, Guido Werdnig,[3] and subsequently confirmed by a German neurologist, Johann Hoffmann, in 1893.[4] Werdnig described "two or more children, who had been well up to that time," who developed a "disease that begins very gradually, in that they cannot use their legs as well as formerly, the children never learn to walk and cannot stand without help. . . . The disease, in a chronic, progressive, centrifugal, and symmetrical course, involves the shoulder girdle, neck and throat muscles, later the muscles of the thigh and arm, then the leg and forearm, and last the muscles of the hands and feet. There is atrophy of the muscles en masse."[3,5]

In 1995, a research group from the Hôpital des Enfants Malades in Paris, France, led by Judith Melki, identified a single mutated gene in SMA, initially referred to as an "SMA-determining gene" and later called survival motor neuron 1, or *SMN1*.[6] In 1999, a study conducted by Christian Lorson and Eric Hahnen in Elliot Androphy's laboratory, as well as by Umrao Monani in Arthur Burghes's laboratory, sought to determine why only the loss of *SMN1*, and not *SMN2*, results in SMA, since the two genes encode identical proteins.[7] The study found that there was a very small difference between *SMN1* and *SMN2*, implying that low levels of the SMN protein produced by *SMN2* were insufficient to protect against the disease's development. Because *SMN2* can produce some SMN protein, however, spinal muscular atrophy is broken down into forms with greater and lesser severity. SMA type 1 is considered the worst type, because patients only have two copies of *SMN2*, versus three or four copies in the less dangerous forms of the disease (also referred to as SMA types 2, 3, and 4).[8]

"In the 80s, 90s, and even in the early 2000s, despite all the interesting work that was being done to characterize the disease,

SMA was still considered a hopeless disease in the clinic, because there was nothing we could do," notes Thomas Crawford, a professor in the department of neurology at the Johns Hopkins University School of Medicine with a research interest in SMA, as well as a practicing physician. "The mission of medical treatment was to try and minimize the complications of weakness."

With rare diseases, such as SMA, that do not have any disease-modifying treatments at the outset and a smaller patient population, it is important to discover the natural history of the disease. Natural history is defined as the normal course of a disease, beginning with the time immediately prior to its inception, progressing through its presymptomatic phase and different clinical stages, and ending at the point where, without external intervention, the patient is either cured, chronically disabled, or dead.[9] This type of understanding about a disease's progression can help greatly when a potential therapeutic candidate shows substantive benefits. Regulatory agencies have demonstrated flexibility when there is "a significant unmet medical need"—that is, "a condition for which there exists no satisfactory method of diagnosis, prevention, or treatment."[10]

A group of doctors and physical therapists, led by Richard Finkel, a neurologist at Nemours Children's Hospital in Orlando, Florida, sought to determine the natural history course of SMA type 1 in babies.[11] The results of this study quantified what doctors already knew: it was a consistently terrible disease. The publication examined "age at death and age at reaching the combined endpoint of either death or requiring at least 16 hours per day of noninvasive ventilation for at least 14 days in the absence of an acute reversible illness or preoperatively (as a surrogate for death)." Of the 34 patients enrolled in the study, early withdrawal occurred for 16 of them, 9 because of death (all within the first 12 months) and 7 for other reasons (including illness and time constraints). The study concluded, "Our data suggest that the probability of reaching a combined endpoint at age 12 months . . . is approximately 50%."

Developmental milestones become groundbreaking, closely monitored events for babies. These include rolling over and sitting up unassisted for a very short period of time. It was almost a forgone conclusion that babies with SMA type 1 would never have the opportunity to take their first steps.

≡ In drug development, having an accurate model on which to test different potential therapies is paramount in advancing through the clinical trial process. Investigators can make a more informed prediction on how a drug will work, even before it is tested in humans. Because SMN2 only differs by less than 1 percent from SMN1, scientists were able to create a mouse model for the disease, referred to as "Delta 7," because of the location of the mutation.[12] "Everything that we needed to be successful fell into place," Crawford recalls. The development of this model also coincided with scientists' growing overall understanding of genetics in the latter half of the twentieth century.[13] This included the discovery and advent of a therapeutic modality (i.e., a form of treatment) called antisense oligonucleuotides.[14,15]

The "central dogma" of molecular biology is the flow of genetic information from DNA to RNA to a functional protein.[16] Think of DNA as a person's way of maintaining an original set of instructions for protein development, which is housed within the nucleus of a cell. RNA serves as a type of copy, or "transcript," of the DNA's instructions, made through a process called transcription. RNA can then move outside the nucleus, in order to guide the process of protein formation, known as translation.

From a drug development perspective, RNA makes an intriguing target, because if DNA contains a mutation, this carries over into RNA. RNA can thus be acted on outside the nucleus. Because RNA is a copy of the original transcript in DNA, manipulating it poses less of a safety risk in introducing a permanent error. Antisense oligonucleotide therapy is made up of nucleic acids that act by binding to RNA and either turning it off completely, so the resulting protein isn't made, or modifying a piece of it that may have a mutation (as happens in SMA), to make a slightly altered protein that works.[17]

Frank Bennett worked for ISIS Pharmaceuticals (now known as Ionis Pharmaceuticals), based in Carlsbad, California. He collaborated with Adrian Krainer, who was at Cold Spring Harbor Laboratory (on Long Island in New York State), to develop an antisense oligonucleotide that could target a sequence known as ISS-N1 and produce functional copies of SMN2 that would potentially yield the missing protein in SMA patients.[18,19] In December 2016, this therapy, after going through clinical trials in SMA patients, became Biogen and Ionis's Spinraza (nusinersen), the first drug in the United States approved by the FDA to treat children and adults with the disease.[20] For their role in the discovery of Spinraza, Bennett and Krainer were co-recipients of a $3 million Breakthrough Prize in 2019. These annual prizes (also referred to as the "Oscars of science") in the life sciences, fundamental physics, and mathematics are awarded through a foundation sponsored by Sergey Brin, Priscilla Chan and Mark Zuckerberg, Ma Huateng, Yuri and Julia Milner, and Anne Wojcicki.[21]

As Crawford notes, "I had previously cared for 72 babies with SMA that died, and making decisions on what [is] the right way to go in terms of care was complicated with no treatment options. The approval of Spinraza and subsequent clinical development programs that have arisen since have been nothing less than transformative. The discussions with families are no longer just 'How do we make this baby's life and the parents' life most fulfilling?' It's 'Which therapeutic approach works best for your family?'"

☰ It is common for there to be less public awareness of rare diseases, but there are several active initiatives to change that. For example, in 2008, EURORDIS (the "voice of rare disease patients in Europe") and its Council of National Alliances launched "Rare Disease Day" to put on events, increase media coverage, and raise awareness about rare diseases among the general public and policy makers.[22] February 28, 2018, was the tenth anniversary of this effort, and the number of participating countries has grown substantially over the years. The development of patient advocacy groups for rare diseases has also been paramount in increased awareness of and resources allocated to treatments and clinical developments. In SMA, a key organization that has played a role in the development of therapies for the disease is Cure SMA. The association directs and invests in comprehensive research to understand and treat the disease, having now raised over $62 million in research funding. Nearly 4,000 families have been helped, and the organization has 115,000 members and supporters throughout the country.[23]

☰ Nicole Almeida ended up contacting Cure SMA, which put the family in touch with its South Florida division. A mom who lived in the area and had a child afflicted with the disease responded. As Nicole recalls, "She said 'I know you're devastated, but here are your options,' and it was relieving to be in touch with someone that understood our position."

From this conversation, the Almeidas learned about Spinraza, which was in clinical trials at the time, as a potential treatment for their son. "We spoke to them [the people at Cure SMA] and Biogen/Ionis had generated clinical data and would've paid for the full trial. It was working, but we understood that the treatments were a lifetime commitment." Spinraza is injected directly into the spinal canal (a process called intrathecal delivery), so that the drug reaches the cerebrospinal fluid. According to the product label, it is administered six times in the first year and then three times in every subsequent year.[24] Nonetheless, as Derwin notes, "We were looking for something bigger, something more permanent."

So the mother Derwin and Nicole met through Cure SMA told them about an early, ongoing clinical trial at Nationwide Children's Hospital in Columbus, Ohio, where a potential one-time gene therapy was being tested. The Almeidas contacted this hospital, and while the doctors there couldn't give them much information at the time about whether the kids receiving this treatment were doing better, they noted that "it is promising." With the due date for Nicole's pregnancy fast approaching, the Almeidas only had a few weeks to make a decision on what course of therapy they would pursue. Their decision to enter the gene therapy trial would prove to be a significant event for not only their family, but also for progress against SMA as a whole.

chapter 4
In Vivo Gene Therapy

Jerry Mendell speaks with the measured pace of a man who has made a career in academia, but his impact on the clinical treatment of children with neuromuscular diseases is second to none. For him, medicine "was an easy decision, it was almost a childhood goal." Similar to Carl June, Mendell was faced with the Vietnam War draft, having graduated from medical school in 1966, completed an internship in neurology at Columbia University in 1967, and finished his residency in 1969. "We had two choices: one was Vietnam, the other was the NIH. . . . I was incredibly relieved to go to the NIH."

Beginning in the 1950s, a "doctor draft" channeled physicians into two years of obligatory service in the US Army, Navy, Air Force, or Public Health Service. For doctors who were interested in research, two programs offered a path to fulfill their military obligation. Frank Berry, the assistant secretary of defense for health and medical affairs, established the first during the Korean

War, in what is known as the Berry Plan physicians could indicate a preference for one of three options:[1]

1. to complete their military service of choice immediately after finishing their internship,
2. to finish one year of residency after their internship, complete their military obligation, and then return to their residency, or
3. to complete their residency training in a specialty of their choice before fulfilling their military obligation.

A physician could also apply to become a commissioned officer in the Public Health Service as part of option 1 and potentially work as a researcher in the NIH's Associate Training Program (ATP), but only a small percentage of those who applied were admitted.[2] When the program began in 1953, only 15 physicians were allowed to join it.[3] In 1960, the Associate Training Program had 68 doctors; in 1965, 153; in 1966, 178; in 1970, 206; and by 1973 (the year Henry Kissinger negotiated a peace settlement in Paris, ending the Vietnam War), 229.

It was an extremely competitive process. As Donald Fredrickson once said, "The best, the absolute cream, the 'Tiffanys,' all applied."[4] Participants in the NIH ATP were nicknamed the "Yellow Berets," a spinoff on the Green Berets, the Special Operations Forces who were considered the best of the best. The academic and medical communities believe that the competitive process to join the Yellow Berets, and the subsequent training they received, prepared them to be the most skilled researchers in the nation.

The Yellow Berets are said to have had a defining influence on academic medicine. A 1998 survey found that 23.6 percent of the professors of medicine at Harvard Medical School and 21 percent at the Johns Hopkins University School of Medicine were former NIH associates.[5] Past participants in the program account for one of every six Nobel laureates in either physiology or medicine between 1985 and 2007, and they make up a similar proportion of members of the National Academy of Sciences within the biomedical fields. Many of NIH's top leaders also had their start in the ATP, including 4 overall directors and 10 institute directors.[5]

In early 1973, having completed his fellowship at the NIH (although he was not part of the Associate Training Program), Mendell began seeking an academic position and found one at Ohio State University. He was able to establish a neuromuscular research program there, where he trained several postdoctoral associates and fellows. Furthermore, Mendell saw the field of gene therapy erupting and established a Center for Gene Therapy at Nationwide Children's Hospital (part of Ohio State University's Department of Pediatrics).

≡ Gene therapy is the process of delivering a working copy of a gene to a patient who has a malfunctioning copy of a gene. This can potentially correct a genetic disease. So how does it work? The process relies on finding a dependable delivery system that can carry the correct gene to the cells that are impacted by it. To find an appropriate vehicle, scientists looked at viruses. Viruses contain a core of RNA or DNA, surrounded by a protein coat. They infect a host cell, where they are able to replicate and grow. In 1953, Wallace Rowe, attempting to isolate the virus that causes the common cold, identified what he called an adenovirus.[6]

In the 1960s, a scientific technique called electron microscopy revealed a simian virus that was contaminating polio vaccines.[7] This led to the discovery of viruses that had the ability to coexist with other viruses—in particular, adenoviruses. Robert Atchison and his colleagues described "small, DNA-containing particles [that] were separated from preparations of simian adenovirus" and suggested that "these adenovirus-associated particles behave as defective viruses."[8] In this paper, Atchison referred to these viruses as adeno-associated viruses, or AAV, a name Wallace Rowe and his colleagues subsequently adopted.[9]

Research in the late 1960s, 1970s, and 1980s began characterizing the composition and active mechanism of both adenoviruses and AAVs in humans.[10] In the 1980s, building on basic research principles developed over the previous 25 years, Nicholas Muzyckza, Jude Samulski, and colleagues were able to clone DNA from AAVs, to facilitate the engineering of recombinant AAVs.[11] This also allowed the process to be scaled up and subsequently used in humans.

In 1990, scientists, researchers, and doctors thought they were ready to test the first application of gene therapy in humans. A 4-year-old girl, Ashanthi (Ashi) DeSilva, became the first patient treated by W. French Anderson, a hematologist at the National Heart, Lung, and Blood Institute,[12] and Michael Blaese at the National Cancer Institute. Ashi had a disease known as adenosine deaminase (ADA) deficiency, which is a condition arising from a mutation in the ADA gene that affects the immune system. This can lead to severe combined immunodeficiency, or SCID.

Patients with SCID have a reduced or absent immune response that leaves them vulnerable to infections, similar to the disease that afflicted the "bubble boy" who had to live in a plastic chamber for protection against diseases. Ashi's treatment involved collecting her blood cells, separating out the T cells, and reengineering them with copies of the ADA gene she lacked, using viruses (known as retroviruses) to deliver the copies. The modified T cells were then grown in petri dishes, until there were enough to treat Ashi.

On September 14, 1990, approximately 1 billion T cells that had been reengineered with a working copy of the ADA gene were infused into Ashi. As Ricki Lewis explains in *The Forever Fix*, "At 12:52 PM, Ken Culver brought in the 'soup'—a pint of murky fluid containing about ten billion of Ashi's corrected white blood cells—and attached the bag to her intravenous line. The infusion took 28 minutes. Ashi received eleven treatments in all, one to two months apart, plus enzyme[s] every week. She had no side effects and started improving after a few infusions.

At the six-month mark, Ashi, her parents, and her two sisters all came down with the flu, and she was the first to recover. That, her mother said, was when they began to look at their daughter as normal."[13] The excitement surrounding the treatment was palpable. In a *New York Times* article, Charles Epstein said, "This is a dramatic event in medical history. Gene therapy is conceptually very profound. We've been waiting years for the day when we could introduce a working gene to replace a gene that doesn't function properly, and I'm delighted it's finally happening."[14]

Did W. French Anderson's gene therapy experiment work? It was hard to say from its small sample size. Siddhartha Mukherjee, in *The Gene*, referred to skeptics of the trial: "Despite Anderson's enthusiasm, and the anecdotal evidence from the families, many proponents of gene therapy . . . were far from convinced that Anderson's trial had amounted to anything more than a publicity stunt."[15] It's probably safe to say that Ashi and her family are convinced that the treatment worked. At the 2018 BIO International Convention held in Boston, Massachusetts, in June, Ashi DeSilva took the stage to a standing ovation from biotechnology industry professionals and said, "I have a message for all of you searching for a treatment and a cure in your lifetime. I hope you can look at my story and know that anything is possible."[16]

The momentum from this trial spurred researchers and doctors alike to dream of the potential for gene therapy to cure diseases with an associated genetic defect, ranging from cancers, to neurological diseases, to heart disease. In this vein, several teams pushed forward in the 1990s to begin gene therapy trials for different genetic diseases, using different types of viruses, such as AAV. In 1999, Mendell's team decided to begin the first gene therapy clinical trial at Nationwide Children's Hospital for a muscular deterioration disorder called limb girdle muscular dystrophy. On September 17, 1999, however, a tragedy involving a young teenager occurred at the University of Pennsylvania. It brought the nascent field to a screeching halt in what has been referred to as the bleakest point in gene therapy's scientific history.[17]

≡ When developing drugs for diseases that have not been treatable before, there is always a risk that a serious adverse event, or even death, can occur. The hope is that an initial focus on safety in its clinical development will mitigate that risk. Jesse Gelsinger was an 18-year-old boy who suffered from a rare metabolic disorder called ornithine transcarbamylase (OTC) deficiency, where a genetic defect in the OTC enzyme prevents the breakdown of proteins. As a result, ammonia begins to accumulate in the body.

Jesse's form of the disease was relatively mild and could be controlled with a low protein diet and a drug regimen of 32 pills per day. According to a *New York Times* article, "He [Jesse] knew when he signed up for the experiment at the University of Pennsylvania that he would not benefit; the study was to test the safety of a treatment for babies with a fatal form of his disorder. Still, it offered hope, the promise that someday Jesse might be rid of the cumbersome medications and diet so restrictive that half a hot dog was a treat."[17]

Similar to Ashi's case with ADA deficiency, OTC deficiency seemed like another ideal candidate to test gene therapy, because the cause of both diseases could be attributed to a single gene mutation. In the OTC case, however, the treatment did not involve extracting blood and reengineering the cells with a virus. The pediatricians running the trial at the University of Pennsylvania were using adenoviruses to deliver the gene directly to cells in the body.

In June 1999, Jesse Gelsinger contacted the University of Pennsylvania team through his local doctors. He and his father, Paul, flew to Philadelphia to meet with Wilson and Mark Batshaw. Jesse returned to Philadelphia to begin the clinical trial and was infused on September 13, 1999. He died 98 hours after receiving the vector (i.e., the adenoviruses carrying the gene), an unexpected event that was subsequently covered in several media outlets and news sources. A *Washington Post* article written on September 29, 1999, noted that "scientists and doctors involved in the case said Gelsinger succumbed over a four-day period after doctors infused a batch of genetically engineered viruses into his liver at the highest dose allowed under an experimental protocol approved by the Food and Drug Administration."[18]

This led to an internal investigation by the University of Pennsylvania, as well as independent hearings in the US Senate and House of Representatives, as well as by Pennsylvania's district attorney, the NIH's Recombinant DNA Advisory Committee (RAC), and the FDA. The FDA suspended the trial, citing its failure to train staff adequately, develop basic operating procedures, and obtain informed consent. In January 2000, the FDA halted the rest of the University of Pennsylvania's trials involving gene therapy and investigated 69 other gene therapy trials in the United States.[19]

In addition, NIH Director Harold Varmus established an Advisory Committee to the Director Working Group on NIH Oversight of Clinical Gene Transfer Research. The committee's report, submitted in July 2000, noted that Jesse "died not as a result of his underlying condition, but seemingly as a direct result of administration of a gene transfer product.... The death of this young man prompted concern about the processes by which gene transfer trials are reviewed, conducted, and monitored by the Food and Drug Administration (FDA) and the National Institutes of Health (NIH), through its Office of Biotechnology Activities (OBA) and its advisory body, the Recombinant DNA Advisory Committee (RAC)."[20]

In an article written nine years after the tragedy, James Wilson, from the University of Pennsylvania, stated, "It became apparent there were shortcomings in several key aspects of the trial; a number of the allegations asserted by the government indeed had merit. This level of non-compliance is inexcusable and as sponsor of the IND [Investigational New Drug protocol] and Director of the Institute for Human Gene Therapy at that time, I accept full responsibility for these problems. I truly believe, however, that the team of physicians, scientists, nurses, and administrative staff that were charged with conducting the clinical trials were an extremely committed and dedicated group of individuals who did the best with what they were provided, and never intended to misrepresent or withhold information."[21]

In *The Gene*, Mukherjee notes Paul Gelsinger's stance: "They didn't have a handle on it [adenovirus] yet . . . they tried it too quickly. They tried it without doing it right. They rushed this thing they really rushed it."[15] The effect Jesse Gelsinger's death had on gene therapy research was clear—until scientists got a true understanding of the safety risks in this treatment, studies would not proceed. "The tragedy was big everywhere," Mendell recalls.[22]

The scientific community had to go back to the drawing board in the mid-2000s to determine the best way to approach gene therapy studies, keeping a clear focus on safety to avoid anything similar to the previous fatal turn of events ever happening again. The promise of providing potential long-term efficacy with just one treatment kept many researchers hopeful that a safer method could be found. As the science began to unfold, AAV vectors seemed to provide the potential for a better benefit-risk profile for patients—enough to warrant attempting human studies again.

"In the 2000s, when there was no funding for gene therapy, it really separated those that were passionate about the science from the 'hangers on,'" notes Katherine High, one of the pioneers in the AAV gene therapy field, who was also at University of Pennsylvania. Using alternative delivery vehicles—given the safety issues with adenoviruses—other groups began reporting promising data with different types of gene therapies for rare diseases. In 2007, AAVs first showed clinical benefits in patients using an *in vivo* (Latin for "performed or taking place in a living organism") method of gene delivery.

That year, groups began clinical trials using a gene called retinal pigment epithelium-specific 65-kD protein, or *RPE65*, for the treatment of a rare form of blindness called Leber's Congenital Amaurosis type 2, or LCA2. This disease is symptomatic, starting in infancy. The eye seemed to be an ideal part of the anatomy to target, because—unlike a systemic delivery, where the treatment can more readily come into contact with the body's immune system—the eye is thought to be "immune privileged."

Three groups began studies. One was a consortium, composed of researchers at the Children's Hospital of Pennsylvania, the University of Pennsylvania, and two Italian institutions: the Telethon Institute of Genetics and Medicine in Pozzuoli, and the Second University of Naples. The second group was a collaboration between teams at the University of Pennsylvania and the University of Florida. The third study was primarily conducted by University College of London. Each of these teams published initial data that showed improvements in visual function, some of which had persisted for one year.[23-25] The gene therapy that the first of the above groups developed was licensed by Spark Therapeutics, a company spun out of the Children's Hospital and led by cofounder and CEO Jeff Marrazzo, with Katherine High joining as cofounder, president, and chief scientific officer.

Following these results, the field began to pick up steam in a clinical setting, with several lessons learned from the past. By using AAVs instead of adenoviruses, the potential toxicity risks were reduced. In 2011, gene therapy hit a major milestone: an impressive result in the treatment of another rare genetic disorder, hemophilia. Hemophilia is a medical condition where an individual's blood does not have the ability to clot. Thus even a slight injury, or simply strenuous exercise, can result in continual bleeding. Hemophilia was first identified in the second century AD in the Babylonian Talmud, when Rabbi Judah decreed, "If she circumcised her first child and he died, and a second one also died, she must not circumcise her third child."[26]

Historically, the disease was also referred to as a "royal disease," due to a large number of descendants of Great Britain's Queen Victoria having the disease.[27] Hemophilia is now identified as an X chromosome–linked genetic disease that affects approximately 20,000 individuals in the United States and potentially more than 400,000 worldwide, according to the National Hemophilia Foundation.[28] Additionally, the disease can be divided into either hemophilia A or hemophilia B, depending on the missing protein that helps with blood clotting: factor VIII for A, and factor IX for B.

The first reported case of hemophilia B was diagnosed in a 10-year-old boy, Stephen Christmas (hence the disease also being known as Christmas disease).[29] At the time, such patients would be disabled before age 20, and their life expectancy averaged 27 years, due to bleeding into vital organs.[30] Initially, patients were given purified forms of the necessary clotting protein, extracted from healthy donors. When these purified clotting factors were used routinely for bleeding episodes, the median lifespan for patients increased to 63 years.[31]

Hemophilia patients began developing HIV, however, which led to an epidemic that was addressed by improved methods for producing factor IX, which involved cloning the relevant gene to reduce the potential for HIV transmission. Another step forward for these patients was the introduction of prophylactic (preventive) therapy instead of on-demand treatment. This was definitively shown to increase the effectiveness of factor replacement therapy.[32] The treatment of hemophilia has subsequently benefited from innovations geared toward reducing the number of treatments for patients, allowing them to continue to live normal lives, free of dangerous bleeding events.

At University College of London, Amit Nathwani added to the thrust of biotechnology innovations for hemophilia by investigating the use of AAV to deliver a functional copy of the missing human factor IX gene *in vivo* to six patients with a severe form of hemophilia B.[33] Such patients have less than 1 percent of the required factor IX protein, whereas the amount of this protein in individuals without hemophilia ranges from 50 to 150 percent.

In another important breakthrough for the field, two patients treated with a low dose achieved a 1 percent level of the factor IX protein, two patients who had a medium dose reached 2.5 percent, and two patients who received a high dose attained an approximate 7 percent level for roughly six months.[34] Importantly, the duration of this benefit has persisted over several years, which has given the field significant hope that gene therapy may provide a one-time treatment for patients with different types of genetic diseases.

Despite all of the clinical trial successes, gene therapy had not been formally approved in any country until 2012, when the European Commission gave its approval to Glybera as a treatment for an ultra-rare inherited disorder called lipoprotein lipase deficiency (LPL).[35] The product works by correcting LPL, enabling muscle cells to produce the enzyme that helps break down fats in the blood, thus reducing the severity of the disease. To obtain regulatory approval, Glybera was studied in 27 patients with LPL who were kept on a low-fat diet. The most common side effect was leg pain from the intramuscular injection of the product.

While Glybera did not succeed as expected commercially,[36] its approval marked the beginning of a viable market for gene therapy. After its approval, Jörn Aldag, the CEO of uniQure BV, the company developing the product, said, "The world has been watching very skeptically, questioning if a gene therapy could ever be approved at all. We have overcome all the barriers and now the European Medicines Agency (EMA) has validated Glybera."[37] As Katherine High recalls, "Glybera's approval showed the gene therapy community that the regulatory agencies were interested in approving products with a positive benefit-risk profile." Small biotechnology companies, such as Spark Therapeutics and bluebird bio, began to gain more notice in the investment community through their gene therapy business models, reinvigorating the hope of treating genetic diseases with a one-time delivery of corrected genes.

≡ After completing his PhD at the Salk Institute in La Jolla, California, Brian Kaspar was recruited by the Center for Gene Therapy, which Jerry Mendell helped establish at Nationwide Children's Hospital. "We took a very systematic approach to test some of the family-tree members of the AAV class," Kaspar notes in a piece recollecting the development of his SMA therapy, adding that "by 2008, we hit upon a virus that had this remarkable capacity to do something we had essentially never seen before."[38]

In 2010, his research group began to see very interesting results in a mouse model of SMA. More specifically, delivery of the *SMN1* gene by a type of AAV called AAV9, which has the ability to target neuronal cells, resulted in 100 percent survival of the mice. This increased the life expectancy from 27 days to over 340 days in mice that normally survived for only 13 days, "highlighting the considerable potential of this method for the treatment of human SMA."[39]

Together, Mendell and Kaspar were able to advance the therapy into a Phase I clinical trial using AAV9 to deliver the *SMN1* gene into three children with SMA.[40] Two weeks after the first patient in the trial was infused with the gene therapy, however, the amount of two liver enzymes—aspartate aminotransferase and alanine aminotransferase, which are associated with inflammation of the liver—was elevated. When there are problems affecting the first patient in a clinical trial, it is very difficult to have faith in trying it with another patient. Mendell went to the FDA and asked, "How should I handle this?"

Luckily, there was a precedent: a corticosteroid therapy called prednisone that was used in the earlier hemophilia trial. Prednisone had lowered the elevated liver enzyme level in the SMN1 trial's initial patient, and Mendell suggested that the next two individuals to be treated would be given prednisone for 24 hours prior to delivery of the gene therapy, and would continue to receive tapered doses of the steroid for the next 30 days. The FDA agreed to this amendment. There were virtually no liver enzyme elevations in the following two patients, allowing the trial to enroll more individuals and increase the dose of the gene therapy.

≡ When babies are born, the first set of tests usually completed on them is called the Apgar Score. The method, developed by Virginia Apgar, rapidly assesses the clinical status of an infant at one and five minutes after birth, with a score of ten indicating "a baby in the best possible condition."[41] When Nicole and Derwin Almeida's son Matteo was delivered, two weeks before the due date, the conversation shifted quickly to when they would be going to Nationwide Children's Hospital to determine if he could be enrolled in the AAV9-SMN1 gene therapy trial.

After doctors again confirmed that Matteo had SMA type 1, on July 25 the family drove to Ohio to begin testing to determine if Matteo met the eligibility criteria. "He was feeding fine and I didn't notice much weakness," Nicole recalls, "but one doctor did notice a bit of neck weakness." During the initial testing period, the Almeidas stayed across the street from Nationwide Children's Hospital. As Derwin notes, "Pretty much through the first month or two of his life, Matteo was a guinea pig."

On August 6, 2015, Matteo received AAV9-*SMN1* gene therapy through an intravenous infusion into his right hand. The whole treatment took about one hour, and he was then transferred to the pulmonary unit. Derwin commented, "Overall, Matteo was fine after the treatment, and we stayed in Ohio for another month, where doctors saw him approximately three times a week. Each visit, we would be in the hospital undergoing different tests for five or six hours a day."

Matteo received his treatment when he was roughly 27 days old, and he was the youngest of the 10 babies who had been given this therapy at the time. Later, the family had to come back to Ohio once a month. Contrary to the natural history of SMA type 1, Matteo began reaching developmental milestones, such as rolling over. "Every time we went, all the treatment staff would come see him," Derwin says. "Even Dr. Mendell is in total awe whenever he sees him." At their two-year appointment, Matteo continued on his path of physical development and was walking all around the hospital, visiting everyone who had ever interacted with him.

When the Almeidas reflect on the treatment's effects on their son, they are quick to give thanks to Jerry Mendell: "We owe our lives to him and his team. Without this therapy we know our lives would be very different." Mendell has been equally humbled by the benefits that have come from Matteo's treatment. At their last appointment, he noted to the Almeidas, "Thank you so much. This validates my life's work."

The therapy was licensed from Nationwide Children's Hospital to AveXis, and Brian Kaspar would join the company as its chief scientific officer. The Phase I study in which Matteo was a participant would go on to enroll a total of 15 patients with SMA type 1. This treatment began to provide additional hope for families with children afflicted with the disease, and it is my second example of a breakthrough.

chapter 5
Sickle Cell Anemia

Terry Jackson was born on July 28, 1973, in Fort Lee, Virginia, where his father was a major in the US Army. The first problems his parents noticed were Terry's swollen hands and feet when he was just a baby, but since sickle cell anemia doesn't show up until fetal hemoglobin is replaced with adult hemoglobin, he wasn't diagnosed with the disease until he was 6 months old. Terry notes, "I don't know life without it. Neither of my parents knew they were carriers, but once I was diagnosed, my mother was very active in learning about the disease. When I would get sick, I would first go to the local army hospital, and if it was bad enough, I would go to the larger hospital in Richmond. The longest I've ever been in the hospital has been 11 days."

In the 1980s, when Terry was receiving treatment for his disease, he became the poster child for the Virginia Sickle Cell Awareness Program (VASCAP), "a statewide program for the education and screening of individuals for the disease of sickle cell anemia or sickle cell trait and for such other genetically related hemoglobinopathies."[1] Terry fondly remembers his summer breaks as a child: "VASCAP had a camp, it was the only day-to-day interaction I had with other people with sickle cell during my childhood." Through the VASCAP program, Terry recalls, "I got to meet the mayor and governor, made appearances to try and raise awareness and money for the disease. In fact, the poster was up right next to school, so my friends understood when I would get sick with VOCs [vaso-occlusive crises]."

Vaso-occlusive crises are one of the most common complications of the disease, and they are a frequent reason for hospitalization. VOCs occur because sickle cell disease distorts red blood cells, forming a crescent shape that inhibits their flow through the blood vessels. The resulting blockages in the vascular system prevent oxygen from reaching bodily tissues, creating severe bouts of pain that are the primary symptom of VOCs. Terry's reaction to the pain from VOCs is variable. At its worst, "it's like an earthquake. There's an epicenter, and then the pain radiates from that point. It can be excruciating and very intense."

During his childhood, Terry felt that he was treated well at the hospital: "It was like a wonderland in pediatrics." When he was in his early 20s, however, he learned that "being an adult patient is so much different than [being] a pediatric patient." For example, a hospital staffer once questioned if he was there solely to get painkilling drugs. "Up until then, I'd never heard anything like that before."

≡ Sickle cell disease impacts approximately 100,000 patients in the United State. As an article from the STAT News website describes, "Racism is a factor—most of the 100,000 U.S. patients with the genetic disorder are African-American—and so is inadequate training of doctors and nurses. And the care is getting worse, sickle cell patients and their doctors said, because the opioid addiction crisis has made ER doctors extremely reluctant to prescribe pain pills."[2] In 2005, the median age of death for sickle cell disease patients was 42 years for females and 38 years for males, with an overall increase in the mortality rate of 0.7 percent each year from 1979 to 2005.[3] The issues in care, moreover, extend beyond life expectancy. For example, in a study conducted by doctors in the Department of Emergency Medicine at Northwestern University's Feinberg School of Medicine, sickle cell patients waited 30 minutes longer to receive pain medication than patients with less severe pain from renal colic.[4]

More than a century after sickle cell anemia was first identified, it still remains a significant unmet medical need. The first reported diagnosis of sickle cell disease in the United States occurred in Chicago in 1910, when physician James Bryan Herrick and his intern, Ernest Irons, found "peculiar elongated and sickle-shaped red blood corpuscles" in their patient, Walter Clement Noel, an African American dentistry student from the island of Grenada who had "jaundice, a history of ulcer of the leg, and severe anemia."[5] After this official documentation of the affliction, other clinicians noted its prevalence among black Americans, although it was unclear why this occurred.

In 1927, E. Vernon Hahn and Elizabeth Biermann Gillespie, from the Laboratory of Surgical Pathology at the Indiana University School of Medicine, published a study that described the scientific data on sickle cell disease to date, noting such qualities as the following:[6]

- It is slowed by cold and accelerated by heat.
- It is independent of exposure to light, but a return of the affected cells to a spherical shape is more rapid in the dark.
- Normal blood cells do not become sickle cells from the serum of a person whose blood contains sickle cells.

By examining a patient who underwent a splenectomy, combined with experiments on the impact of different gases, Hahn and Gillespie discovered that the crescent shape of red blood cells in sickle cell anemia patients was due to a loss of oxygen.

≡ Linus Pauling was born in Portland, Oregon, on February 28, 1901, to druggist Herman Henry William Pauling and Lucy Isabelle Darling. He attended public elementary and high schools and graduated from Oregon State College with a bachelor's degree in chemical engineering. He completed his graduate studies at the California Institute of Technology (Caltech), where he was awarded a PhD in chemistry, with minors in physics and math. In 1927, he joined the Caltech faculty and conducted research on the formation of chemical bonds. Pauling is also known for his wide-ranging research interests. He even hypothesized that a gene might consist of two mutually complementary strands,[7,8] a concept that James Watson and Francis Crick verified in their discovery of the structure of DNA in 1953. Pauling won the Nobel Prize in Chemistry in 1954 and the Nobel Peace Prize in 1962.

During the mid-1930s, part of Pauling's research interests shifted to the field of biochemistry and were funded by the Rockefeller Foundation. In 1934, he investigated hemoglobin, the protein in red blood cells that is responsible for transporting oxygen in the blood. In New York City in 1945, Pauling attended a committee meeting, composed of doctors appointed by President Franklin D. Roosevelt, on the topic of medical research in the United States.[9] He was in the audience at an informal after-dinner presentation by William Castle, a physician and professor of medicine at Harvard University. Castle noted that the shape of red blood cells in patients with sickle cell disease differed, based on the whether the cell was in the arteries or the veins. This is where Pauling first learned about sickle cell anemia.

In a 1960 interview, he recalled what happened that night, when he wondered, "Could it be possible that this disease, which seems to be a disease of the red cell because the red cells in the patients are twisted out of shape, could [it] really be a disease of the hemoglobin molecule? . . . 'Well,' I said to the man who was talking about the disease [Dr. Castle], 'has anyone ever suggested that this might be a disease of the hemoglobin molecule?' And he said, 'Not so far as [he'd] ever heard.' And I said, 'Do you think it would be alright if I were to look at this hemoglobin from these patients and see?' And he said, 'I don't see why not.'"[10]

On November 6, 1946, Pauling wrote to Castle, stating, "I now have a graduate student (Harvey Itano, M.D.) beginning work on the problem of the relation between the nature of the hemoglobin in sickle cell anemia and the phenomenon of sickling."[11] Itano, an American citizen of Japanese heritage, was born in California. He attended the St. Louis University School of Medicine and learned of Linus Pauling through a chapter the latter wrote in a medical textbook.

In 1949, Pauling, Itano, S. J. Singer, and Ibert C. Wells published an article in *Science*, suggesting that the sickling of red blood cells occurred because of an error in the hemoglobin gene inside the cells.[12] Later investigations determined that the disease could be pinpointed to a single mutation in hemoglobin, and it became the focus of multiple researchers, ranging from molecular biologists to pediatricians to cardiologists. From a scientific perspective, sickle cell anemia represents a window into understanding the role that identifying the drivers of a disease can play in finding potential cures.

In the 1950s, British researcher A. C. Allison suggested that the sickle cell abnormality in the hemoglobin gene persisted because "it protected its carriers against some other fatal disease—say malaria."[13] Therefore, the hereditary nature of the disease brought a different viewpoint on sickle cell anemia to those studying it. Pauling became a proponent of genetic counseling, which later evolved into his public campaign to support eugenics for alleviating human suffering.[14]

Eugenics is the science of "improving" a human population by controlled breeding, in order to increase the occurrence of desirable heritable characteristics, whether it be removing disease or adding advantageous features. These topics have always led to significant ethical debates. In the late 1960s, Pauling once said, "I have suggested that the time might come in the future when information about heterozygosity [inheriting different forms of a particular gene from each parent] in such serious genes as the sickle cell anemia gene would be tattooed on the forehead of the carriers, so that young men and women would at once be warned not to fall in love with each other."[15]

While attempting to arrest the spread of genetic disease, he also incited a plethora of detractors, due to the racial and social undertones of what he was advocating, because sickle cell anemia overwhelmingly impacts the African American population. Pauling later abandoned this view. The social and political implications of sickle cell anemia, however, remain interconnected with the disease in America.

☰ Sickle cell anemia reached the status of a national symbol in 1971–1972. As Keith Wailoo explains in *Dying in the City of Blues: Sickle Cell Anemia and the Politics of Race and Health*, "Its public image reflected the political realities confronting African Americans. To understand the new face of sickle cell anemia, it is crucial to understand the rise of black political clout in the wake of the Voting Rights Act of 1965, to examine how the disease experience became [a] cultural symbol for liberal Americans, and to explore the response of conservatives to the disease's celebrity and political significance."[16]

By October 1971, bills calling for the allocation of as much as $600 million for sickle cell anemia research were introduced in both the US House of Representatives and the Senate.[17,18] John Tunney of California addressed the Senate floor and discussed the prevalence of this disease, compared with others, and the disparity in funding for it, noting that "in 1967, there were an estimated 1,155 new cases of sickle cell anemia, 1,206 of cystic fibrosis, 813 of muscular dystrophy, and 350 of phenylketonuria [a rare inherited disorder that causes an amino acid called phenylalanine to build up in the body]. Yet in 1968, volunteer organizations raised $1.9 million for cystic fibrosis, $7.9 million for muscular dystrophy, but only $50,000 for sickle cell research."[18]

On May 16, 1972, President Richard Nixon signed the National Sickle Cell Anemia Control Act into law, noting that "in February 1971, I pledged that this Administration would reverse the record of neglect on this dread disease."[19] Nixon also stated that in fiscal 1972, $10 million was used to expand sickle cell programs, a tenfold budget increase over fiscal 1971. Moreover, Nixon added, in his March 1972 health message, he proposed to raise the funding level of sickle cell anemia activities for fiscal 1973 to $15 million, as well as to expand the Veterans Administration's sickle cell program. Nixon concluded his address by saying, "The National Sickle Cell Anemia Control Act, which I am today signing, follows the course that we have charted. These actions make clear, I believe, the urgency with which this country is working to alleviate and arrest the suffering from this disease."

☰ In the early 1980s, a cancer drug called 5-azacytidine was able to increase fetal hemoglobin (HbF), a type of hemoglobin that is produced in infancy and is also more resistant to sickling, compared with adult hemoglobin. In a study that treated a patient with 5-azacytidine, the amount of HbF rose from 1.8 percent to 8.9 percent. This was accompanied by an increase in peripheral blood hemoglobin concentration, going from a density of 8 grams per deciliter (g/dL) to 12 g/dL. (The normal density of hemoglobin in men is approximately 13.5 g/dL to 17.5 g/dL.)[20] These results generated some hope of a transformative therapy, with popular media reports seizing on the potential of increasing a patient's HbF in treating sickle cell anemia.[21] Unfortunately, these benefits came with toxic side effects that showed 5-azacytidine had the potential to cause cancer in laboratory animals.[22]

Due to concerns about the toxicity of 5-azacytidine, the Bristol Myers pharmaceutical company developed hydroxycarbomide (otherwise known as hydroxyurea), a chemotherapeutic drug used in nonmalignant diseases such as sickle cell anemia, as a safer alternative. Preliminary studies with hydroxyurea in 10 hospitalized patients, conducted at the National Institutes of Health and Johns Hopkins University, resulted in 70 percent of these patients responding positively to the drug, with a 2- to 10-fold increase in fetal hemoglobin, after being treated for three months.[23]

The results led to additional major media reports on the trial, with the *New York Times* commenting that this experimental drug treatment "may be the first to affect the disorder itself and not just the symptoms."[24] The doctors who conducted the initial *New England Journal of Medicine* study were cautious about the results, however, with its chief author, Griffin Rodgers, noting in the *New York Times* article, "We would suggest that the drug not be used by practicing physicians until we know more about optimal doses. . . . [Doctors] who think their patients might benefit should try getting them into clinical trials where dosages can be carefully monitored."[24] This drives home a larger point in pharmaceutical development—namely, that earlier results must be viewed cautiously until they are verified in larger studies.

A study in 1995, using a more optimal trial design with a placebo control group, enrolled 148 men and 151 women at 21 clinics and tested the ability of hydroxyurea to reduce the frequency of painful crises in adults with a history of three or more such crises per year.[25] The clinical trial was halted after only 21 months of study, instead of the initially planned 24 months, due to its significant success: a 44 percent reduction in the median annual rate of VOCs that the authors deemed "both clinically meaningful and statistically significant." Additionally, the trial saw reductions in the number of transfusions and the frequency of acute chest syndrome (chest pain, cough, fever, low oxygen level, and abnormal substances in the lungs), both of which are complications related to the disease.

These promising results were not without safety concerns about the drug, with physicians noting that the excitement over a potentially effective pharmacologic intervention in sickle cell anemia "should not obscure the need for caution with [the] use of hydroxyurea in this setting and for continued monitoring for secondary malignant conditions in patients treated for long periods."[26] They were warning that the potential benefits of hydroxyurea must be weighed against the potential risks of secondary neoplasms (cancers arising in an individual as a result of previous chemotherapy or radiation therapy). In the late 1990s, regulatory approval of hydroxyurea provided the first FDA-approved therapy to reduce the frequency of painful VOCs and the need for blood transfusions in adult patients with sickle cell anemia whose crises were moderate to severe.[27]

In recent years, more capital investments in sickle cell disease therapeutics are leading to new treatment options. In 2017, the FDA approved the use of Endari, from Emmaus Life Sciences, to reduce the acute complications of sickle cell disease in adult and pediatric patients five years of age and older. It was the second drug to receive accreditation to treat this affliction since the discovery of the disease over 100 years ago, with confirmation coming more than 20 years after hydroxyurea's certification.[28] In 2019, Novartis's Adakveo, which diminishes the frequency of vaso-occlusive crises in adults and pediatric patients aged 16 years and older with sickle cell disease, received FDA accreditation.[29] The FDA also used its accelerated approval pathway in 2019 to ratify the use of Oxbryta, an oral therapy developed by Global Blood Therapeutics to increase hemoglobin levels and decrease end organ damage (damage occurring in major organs fed by the circulatory system).[30]

Currently, the only approved "curative" therapy for sickle cell disease is a hematopoietic stem cell transplant, employing cells usually derived from bone marrow, peripheral (whole) blood, or umbilical cord blood. A suitable donor must be found, however, and even then there are substantial risks with this therapy. With a large US population suffering from sickle cell anemia, and an estimated 20 million patients worldwide, accelerating disease-modifying therapies for it remains a key goal for patients, families, and communities.

chapter 6
Ex Vivo Gene Therapy

M arina Cavazzana studied medicine in Padua, Italy, and received her MD degree in 1983. She then earned a certification in pediatrics in 1987 and a PhD in life sciences in 1993, both at Université Paris VII. During her training in pediatrics, she learned the technique for hematopoietic (blood) stem cell transplants. This procedure consists of placing healthy bone marrow (usually from a sibling) into children afflicted with bloodborne diseases. It was initially used for patients with Fanconi anemia, a rare inherited disorder that leads to bone marrow failure.[1]

In the mid-1990s, she began investigating gene therapy as a way to potentially mitigate some of the side effects of transplants, such as graft-versus-host disease, which is particularly severe when a compatible donor can't be found. The focus of her gene therapy research was on taking a patient's defective bone marrow cells and "correcting" (i.e., modifying) them outside the body, in an *ex vivo* process (Latin for "out of the living [organism]"). This technique employs a gamma-retrovirus, a different type of virus from AAV, that can convert its RNA into DNA using an enzyme called reverse transcriptase. This enzyme allows the virus's DNA to be integrated directly into the DNA of a host cell. (While the HIV virus is a retrovirus, the first vector, or delivery mechanism, used in Cavazzana's studies was a different virus).

In 2000, following the 1999 death of Jesse Gelsinger in a gene therapy trial at the University of Pennsylvania (see chapter 4), Cavazzana and her colleagues in the Unité d'Immunologie et d'Hématologie Pédiatriques at Hôpital Necker in Paris, France, published a study in *Science* reporting the first clinical benefit of a gene therapy for children afflicted by severe combined immunodeficiency-X1, or SCID-X1, a genetic disease characterized by a disorder in the immune system.[2] As W. F. Anderson noted in an accompanying perspective section in that issue of *Science*, the "encouraging new results . . . have brought cautious optimism back to the gene therapy field."[3] This initial success led to gene-corrected bone marrow cells being reintroduced into five boys with X chromosome–linked severe combined immunodeficiency, with four out of the five showing a "clear-cut clinical improvement."[4]

Unfortunately, a later paper noted that one of the 10 patients in the first French clinical trial had developed leukemia about two years after receiving a gene transfer.[5] This first report of a negative consequence in gene-corrected therapy has since been followed by five others. France's National Agency for the Safety of Medicine and Health Products (Agence Nationale de Sécurité du Médicament et des Produits de Santé, or ANSM) and the US Food and Drug Administration, suspended trials using retroviral vectors to insert genes into defective cells, while The UK Department of Health and Social Care's Gene Therapy Advisory Committee recommended that additional measures be put in place to protect patients undergoing gene therapy trials.[6] Similar to what happened for *in vivo* gene therapy with adenoviruses, the field of *ex vivo* gene-corrected therapies went back to the drawing board and rebounded with a type of self-inactivating virus that did not produce the side effects seen in the initial clinical trials using the first generation of vectors.[5]

≡ In 2010, *ex vivo* gene therapy had a major breakthrough with the report of positive results in a patient with beta-thalassemia.[7] Beta-thalassemia is a blood disorder that reduces the production of hemoglobin and requires recurrent blood transfusion therapy. In the study, an adult patient was treated with a lentiviral vector (a type of retrovirus) that contained the missing gene in his blood and subsequently did not need transfusions for more than 7 years. One of the study's authors, Philippe Leboulch, noted, "For beta-thalassemia, we have worked intensely for almost 20 years to design, develop and manufacture this treatment to provide a sustained high level hemoglobin production, resulting in a major clinical benefit. It has been very rewarding to follow this patient as his life has dramatically improved since receiving our treatment."[8]

Sickle cell anemia arises from a single gene mutation. Due to proof of effective *ex vivo* gene correction for this disease in mouse models,[9] and the success of this therapy for patients with beta-thalassemia, in 2014 a boy with sickle cell anemia was treated with a lentiviral vector containing the corrected form of the mutated gene.[10] The procedure was done via an autologous hematopoietic stem cell transplant performed at the Department of Biotherapy in Necker Children's Hospital in Paris. The boy was diagnosed with sickle cell anemia at birth and had been given hydroxyurea therapy between the ages of 2 and 9, but this treatment was unable to significantly reduce his symptoms. In 2010, he received blood transfusions, after having had an average of 1.6 VOCs annually in the nine years before the transfusions began. He underwent his last transfusion 88 days after the cell transfer, which resulted in stable hemoglobin levels. Moreover, more than 15 months after receiving gene therapy, the boy, who was now a teenager, had not experienced any disease-related symptoms and stopped taking all medications, including pain medicines.

The lentiviral *ex vivo* gene therapy was licensed by a firm called bluebird bio, which is evaluating the safety and effectiveness of the product, now called LentiGlobin BB305.[11] At the 2018 European Hematology Association's annual meeting in Stockholm, Sweden, the company presented early data from a refined manufacturing process. Julie Kanter, a lead investigator in the Phase I study, noted that the early data "are very exciting and provide increasing confidence that LentiGlobin has the potential to deliver transformative benefit to patients."[12] At the 2020 European Hematology Association's annual meeting, LentiGlobin BB305 showed a near-complete reduction (99.5 percent mean reduction) in VOCs for 14 patients, after at least six months of follow-up. Kanter stated, "The promising results of this study, which show patients have an almost complete elimination of VOCs and ACS [acute chest syndrome], suggest LentiGlobin for SCD has real potential to provide a significant impact for people living with sickle cell disease."[13]

Unfortunately, in February 2021, the FDA placed a clinical hold on the sickle cell program, due to a reported SUSAR, or suspected unexpected serious adverse reaction, in a patient in the clinical trial who developed acute myeloid leukemia.[14] A subsequent analysis of this patient determined that it was very unlikely the case was related to the BB305 lentiviral vector. In June 2021, the FDA lifted its clinical hold on the program, although the negative event underscores its potential risks.

Other approaches to generating *ex vivo* gene therapies to treat sickle cell disease and ameliorate vaso-occulsive events are in progress. One of these approaches, called CTX001—being codeveloped by CRISPR Therapeutics, in collaboration with Vertex Pharmaceuticals—is the first use of CRISPR/Cas9 technology in patients. It involves editing a patient's hematopoietic stem cells to knock out a gene, which would allow an increase in fetal hemoglobin, and then reinfusing the corrected cells back into the patient.[15] As I mentioned in the previous chapter, HbF is the protein that fetuses make in the womb to extract oxygen from their mother's blood. Once a baby is born, fetal hemoglobin, or HbF, is replaced by adult hemoglobin. Infants carrying the defective gene become symptomatic as the adult sickling hemoglobin becomes more prevalent. In patients where HbF persists into adulthood, however, little or no disease is seen.

In 1987, Japanese scientists studying the bacteria *E. coli* came across repeating sequences in its DNA but wrote that their "biological significance is unknown."[16] Other researchers, such as Francisco Mojica, who was working on his PhD in Spain, found similar DNA sequences in ancient archea (a single-cell organism with similarities to bacteria). These were repeated up to 600 times in a row and eventually became known as clustered regularly interspaced short palindromic repeats, or CRISPR.[17]

In 2007, scientists studying *Streptococcus* showed that these clusters were part of the bacteria's immune system, providing resistance against viruses.[18] When an infection occurs, the bacteria being attacked produce an enzyme, called Cas9, to neutralize the virus. In 2012, researchers, led by Jennifer Doudna at the University of California Berkley and Dr. Emanuelle Charpentier at Umeå University in Sweden, published a landmark paper in *Science* that identified the CRISPR/Cas9 system's ability to be programmed to cut out a genome at any site of interest, which has the potential to permanently alter DNA.[19] This discovery lead to Doudna and Charpentier winning the 2020 Nobel Prize in Chemistry. Following this initial discovery, it was shown that CRISPR/Cas9 could be used to edit the genomes of mouse or human cells.[20]

CRISPR/Cas9 technology could have far-reaching ramifications, including the potential to cure disease, but "some research has hinted that CRISPR's off-target effects warrant greater attention."[21] Nonetheless, it is unlikely to create the supersized, uncontrollable crocodiles and wolves featured in the 2018 movie *Rampage*, starring Dwayne "The Rock" Johnson.[22]

According to Doudna, "As long as the genetic code for a particular trait is known, scientists can use CRISPR to insert, edit, or delete the associated gene in virtually any living plant's or animal's genome.... Practically overnight, we have found ourselves on the cusp of a new age in genetic engineering and biological mastery—a revolutionary era in which the possibilities are limited only by our collective imagination."[23] CRISPR/Cas9 has become the latest in a class of gene-editing technologies, and it is likely to lead to several more breakthroughs in the coming years, due to its ease of use and relatively low cost.

≡ On July 2, 2019, Victoria Gray, a 34-year-old mother of three who first experienced symptoms of sickle cell anemia when she was 3 months old, underwent the first infusion of *ex vivo* CRISPR-edited stem cells. Her journey, chronicled by NPR, involved an infusion of over 2 billion modified cells and a hospital stay lasting almost two months.[24] A paper delivered at the 2020 American Society of Hematology's annual meeting presented data from three sickle cell disease patients treated with CTX001, including Victoria Gray, with follow-ups ranging from 3 to 15 months.[25]

Heading into the presentation, it was thought that the measure of success in ameliorating symptoms of the disease would be roughly 30 percent. Instead, the median percentage of fetal hemoglobin was 10 g/dL (37 percent) three months after the transfusion in all the patients, 11.4 g/dL (48 percent) after six months in two patients, and 12 g/dL (43 percent) after 15 months in the first treated patient. Significantly, the latter three patients had been VOC-free for 3.8, 7.8, and 16.6 months, respectively, a marketed reduction from their previous average annual VOC rates of 4, 7.5, and 7.

Updated data from CTX001, presented at the 2021 European Hematology Association's meeting, continued to show benefits in a greater number of patients.[26] In seven treated individuals, the mean percentage of fetal hemoglobin was 37 percent 3 months after the transfusion, 45 percent after 6 months, and 42 percent after 21 months, with no VOCs since the CRISPR/Cas9 treatment.

In patients with beta-thalassemia (a disease with similarities to sickle cell anemia) who were also treated with CTX001, 15 of them showed increases in their fetal hemoglobin. They, too, no longer needed blood transfusions, which are a current standard-of-care for people with beta-thalassemia. In chapter 12, I will discuss the potential breakthroughs that could be catalyzed by gene editing.

≡ Terry Jackson has a hard time remembering how many clinical trials he's been enrolled in thus far, because "I've been in so many. They come to the emergency room, you sign a waiver, they collect your blood, and then they're gone and you never see them again." He's found some success with blood transfusion therapy and a lower dose of hydroxyurea to help mitigate the disease's complications, and he was able to overcome the obstacles presented by his illness to obtain his PhD.

When you ask Terry about the potential for finding a cure for sickle cell disease, he can only say, "Of course I want the disease to be cured, but most of all I want people with sickle cell to have a better overall quality of life. My friend is 21 years old and wants to be a scientist also, but she's in the hospital all the time and has had to drop out of school because of her complications." He's also spoken to the global community of sickle cell sufferers in places such as Africa or the West Indies, where they may not yet have the means to receive a complex therapy, such as a hematopoietic stem cell transplant.

Marina Cavazzana echoes this sentiment: "I hope that, over time, there is the development of a more automatized process that will allow application of technology to the greatest number of patients." In the scientific and medical realms, the combination of an understanding of sickle cell disease and innovations in genetic and cellular medicines has resulted in my third example of a breakthrough. While *ex vivo* gene therapies are at an earlier stage than my previous two examples of breakthroughs in medicine, there remains hope that time and technological advancements in the manufacture and design of these treatments will yield a cure for sickle cell anemia.

≡ The regulatory process in biotechnology is its most unique attribute, compared with practices in other industries. A product must have a positive benefit-risk profile in order to gain approval for commercial use. This is a necessary mitigating factor, where proper precautions must be balanced against the desire to quickly get medicines into the hands of physicians and patients. In the following chapters, I outline a brief history of pharmaceutical regulation and show how each of this book's examples of breakthroughs in medicine reached their respective milestones of regulatory approval.

chapter 7
A Brief History of FDA Regulations

n 1906, President Theodore Roosevelt signed the Food and Drug Act (also known as the Wiley Act, named after Harvey Washington Wiley, the chief chemist for the Bureau of Chemistry in the US Department of Agriculture) into law, thereby creating what would be known officially in 1930 as the US Food and Drug Administration, or FDA. The impact of Upton Sinclair's novel, *The Jungle*, contributed to public interest in the development of the FDA.[1,2] His book detailed unsanitary working conditions and unscrupulous practices in the meatpacking industry, exposing the public to a graphic depiction of disease-ridden and contaminated meat.

An important piece of legislation for the FDA's current jurisdiction is the 1938 Food, Drug, and Cosmetic Act. Drafting of the original bill began in late March 1933, and on December 7 and 8, 1933, the first hearings were scheduled. One complaint from the drug industry at the time was that the bill would "deprive the American people of their right to 'self-medication.'" The FDA's strategy to counter this stance was to assemble exhibits illustrating how the current law was ineffective and could negatively impact consumers. The displays, dubbed a "Chamber of Horrors" by a columnist who visited the exhibit, included "pictures, labels, and advertisements of ineffective or harmful and occasionally lethal nostrums, dangerous cosmetic preparations, and adulterated or deceptively packaged and labeled foodstuffs," effectively communicating these issues to the public.[3]

While debate on the legislation was underway, including President Franklin D. Roosevelt's statement to Congress in support of the bill,[4] Archie Shepherd Calhoun of Mt. Olive, Mississippi, was prescribing a drug—elixir sulfanilamide, produced by the S. E. Massengill Company—to his patients. It was manufactured using a toxic chemical—diethylene glycol, or DEG—as a solvent. Calhoun was a well-respected physician who, by the late 1930s, had practiced for over 26 years. In a photo published on November 8, 1937, in *Life* magazine, he is dressed in a three-piece suit, complemented by horn-rimmed glasses—an outfit befitting a physician of the time—with his eyes cast downward.[5]

The S. E. Massengill Company was founded in 1897 by Normal Hood Massengill and Dr. Samuel Evans Massengill, with a main research and production facility in Bristol, Tennessee, that employed over 200 people. Sulfanilamide was one of the first antibiotics, proven to be an effective treatment for streptococcal infections (e.g., strep throat and scarlet fever).[6] A Massengill salesman convinced the company that clients wanted a liquid formulation. The company's chief pharmacist at the time, Harold Cole Watkins, approved the use of DEG without any toxicity tests (since none were required). The company did test the mixture for flavor, appearance, and fragrance, however, eventually adding a raspberry flavoring to enhance its taste.

Elixir sulfanilamide ended up being responsible for the deaths of more than 100 people in 15 states, due to the addition of DEG in the mixture. Six of Calhoun's patients died, and seven others suffered "varying degrees of mental and physical torture" but eventually recovered. In a letter explaining the tragedy, written to President Roosevelt on October 22, 1937, Calhoun stated, "Nobody but Almighty God and I can know what I have been through these past few days. I have been familiar with death in the years since I received my M.D. from Tulane University School of Medicine. . . . Any doctor who has practiced more than a quarter of a century has seen his share of death." He then continued, "But to realize that six human beings, all of them my patients, one of them my best friend [Reverend J. E. Byrd, secretary of the Mississippi Baptist Board], are dead because they took medicine that I prescribed for them innocently, and to realize that that medicine which I had used for years in such cases suddenly had become a deadly poison in its newest and most modern form, as recommended by a great and reputable pharmaceutical firm in Tennessee: well, that realization has given me such days and nights of mental and spiritual agony as I did not believe a human being could undergo and survive. I have known hours when death for me would be a welcome relief from this agony."

The outcry from this public health disaster propelled the bill through Congress, and President Roosevelt signed the Food, Drug, and Cosmetic Act on June 25, 1938. Under this act, the primary focus of the FDA's drug approval process was to ensure that the products were safe for humans. In clinical developments today, safety thresholds remain the key factor in determining whether a potential drug candidate progresses to later-stage trials.[7]

≡ Chemie Grünenthal GmbH developed the drug thalidomide in the 1950s, initially as an anticonvulsive in the treatment of epileptic seizures, but it also made its users sleepy. During the research process, animal testing did not reveal any lethal dose of drug.[8] Thalidomide was first commercialized in 1957 as an over-the-counter product that was completely safe for use with sleeping issues. The drug was seen as harmless, even during pregnancy, and was used to relieve morning sickness, making it popular with pregnant women.[9] (This was also a time when drugs were not thought to cross over from the mother's body into the placenta). By 1960, 46 countries marketed thalidomide, with an estimated 14.6 tons sold in Germany, and sales that were on par with Bayer aspirin.

In 1961, William McBride, an Australian obstetrician, published a letter to the editor in *The Lancet* that began, "In recent months I have observed that the incidence of multiple severe abnormalities in babies delivered of women who were given the drug thalidomide ('Distaval') during pregnancy, as an anti-emetic or as a sedative, to be almost 20 percent. . . . Have any of your readers seen similar abnormalities in babies delivered of women who have taken this drug during pregnancy?"[10]

Around this same time, Widukind Lenz, a German pediatrician and geneticist, made independent observations in the children of patients being treated with thalidomide.[11] He had noted an outbreak of limb and ear malformation in Western Germany between November 11 and 16, 1961, and contacted Chemie Grünenthal. After ten days of discussions with the company, the drug was withdrawn in Germany but continued to be sold in other countries, such as Belgium, Brazil, Canada, Italy, and Japan.

In a speech given several years later, Lenz noted that if thalidomide is taken during a sensitive period in pregnancy (between days 35 and 49), various malformations can occur, including no ears, the absence of arms, phocomelia (a deformity in which the hands or feet are attached close to the trunk, with underdeveloped or absent limbs), hands with three fingers, and thumbs with three joints. He estimated that approximately 40 percent of thalidomide victims died before their first birthday. It has since been ascertained that the original catastrophe disfigured roughly 20,000 babies and killed 80,000, although it is unclear how many miscarriages the drug caused.[12] Survivors had early onset arthritis and chronic pain, driving them to rely on their parents and family members, social benefits or health insurance payments, or charity. Many have been forced into early retirement.

In 1960, the Richardson-Merrell Company applied to the FDA for approval to sell thalidomide in the United States, under the trade name Kevadon, hoping to market it over the counter to treat alcoholism, anorexia, asthma, cancer, "poor schoolwork," premature ejaculation, and tuberculosis.[13] Frances Kelsey, a physician and pharmacologist at the FDA, received the application. He noticed the reports of what was happening in Germany and requested more information. At the same time, Senator Estes Kefauver of Tennessee introduced a bill to enhance the safety regulations on drugs, independent of Richardson-Merrell's submission to the FDA. Kefauver learned about thalidomide's effects from an article by Helen Taussig, published in *Scientific American* in 1962, that discussed the drug's synthesis, distribution, and resulting toxicity.[14] Importantly, Taussig noted that she was convinced the US regulatory systems would have approved thalidomide for widespread distribution.

The public health tragedy of thalidomide galvanized Congress into passing the Kefauver-Harris Amendments to the 1938 Food, Drug, and Cosmetic Act.[13] The 1962 amendments required drug manufacturers to prove the effectiveness of the drugs distributed on the US market, as well as their safety. The amendments also stated that the FDA had to approve a new drug application (NDA) before that company could commercialize the product. Opponents of the amendments made the argument that the efficacy requirements would raise the price of drugs, increase research and development costs, discourage drug development, and remove a consumer's personal choice on whether to use a drug. Prior to the amendments, the FDA was approving an average of 46.2 new drugs annually. In the following decade, this number dropped to 15.7.

≣ In the 1990s, when FDA backlogs in the drug approval process delayed the marketing launch of many drugs, a number of patient groups with devastating diseases expressed their frustration. Once more, the underlying driver was a current public health crisis—this time, the AIDS epidemic.[15] On June 5, 1981, the US Centers for Disease Control and Prevention (CDC) published a report describing cases of a rare lung infection, *Pneumocystis carinii* pneumonia (PCP), in five young, previously healthy gay men in Los Angeles, California.[16] Within days, the CDC received numerous reports of similar cases of infections, including Kaposi's sarcoma (a rare and aggressive cancer), among gay men in New York and California.

The saga of the AIDS epidemic continued throughout the 1980s, which included the story of Ryan White, a 13-year-old hemophiliac who was diagnosed with AIDS as a result of a blood transfusion and subsequently barred from school in Indiana. On March 20, 1987, the FDA approved azidothymidine, or AZT, an antiviral drug made by the Burroughs Wellcome Company under the brand name Retrovir. Daniel Carpenter, in his book *Reputation and Power: Organizational Image and Pharmaceutical Regulation at the FDA*, details the FDA's regulatory process, which includes an advisory panel of key opinion leaders (trusted, well-respected individuals with proven experience and expertise in a particular field) from academia, government, and industry.[17] Ellen Cooper was the FDA's top AIDS drug regulator at the time. According to Carpenter, "Throughout her observation of clinical trials and her review, Cooper was thoroughly aware of her several audiences," and "she knew that she was making history, not just for the fantastic and legendary variety (reviewing the first drug submitted for a global health epidemic), but of the juridical sort.

Cooper foresaw that her procedures and recommendations would have 'major implications for the testing and evaluation of other drugs in AIDS.'" In approving the drug, there was some subjectivity introduced into the language of "adequate and well-controlled investigations" that was part of the Kefavauer-Harris Amendments.

In the late 1980s, activist organizations accused the FDA of delaying the approval of medications to fight HIV. They staged large protests, with the goal of speeding up the drug regulatory review process. On October 11, 1988, an activist group, the AIDS Coalition to Unleash Power (ACT-UP), organized a protest. It began with a rally at the US Department of Health and Human Services, under a banner stating "Health Care Is Right," and proceeded the following morning to FDA headquarters in Washington, DC.

According to Douglas Crimp, AIDS activists prepared an "FDA Action Handbook," conducted a series of teach-ins for ACT-UP members, and presented the information to the press.[18] As he noted, "The FDA action was 'sold' in advance to the media almost like a Hollywood movie, with a carefully prepared and presented press kit, hundreds of phone calls to members of the press, and activists' appearances scheduled on television and radio talk shows around the country."

When the demonstration took place, the media were not only there to get the story, they knew what that story was, and they reported it with a degree of accuracy and sympathy." Demands to the FDA included shortening the drug approval process; getting rid of double-blind, placebo-controlled trials; including people from all affected populations, at all stages of HIV infection, in clinical trials; requiring Medicaid or private health insurers to pay for experimental drug therapies; and insisting the FDA support community groups working to keep their members alive.

The newfound voice of the activist community, catalyzed by the AIDS epidemic, led to increased collaboration between advocates, regulators, and industry. It also resulted in legislation, such as the Prescription Drug User Fee Act (PDUFA) in 1992, to supplement the FDA budget outside of direct appropriations from Congress. In December 1992, the FDA also created an accelerated approval mechanism that applied to new drug products, allowing the agency "to base accelerated approval for drugs for serious conditions that fill an unmet medical need on whether the drug has an effect on a surrogate or an intermediate clinical endpoint."[19]

A surrogate endpoint allowed drugs to be developed if they showed "a marker . . . that is thought to predict clinical benefit [i.e., a positive therapeutic effect that is clinically meaningful in the context of a given disease], but is not itself a measure of clinical benefit. Likewise, an intermediate clinical endpoint is a measure of a therapeutic effect that is considered reasonably likely to predict the clinical benefit of a drug, such as an effect on irreversible morbidity and mortality." This accelerated process also permitted the FDA to approve an effective drug that could only be administered safely if its distribution or use were restricted.[20]

This pathway has led to expedited therapies for patients as well as controversy. In 2001, after FDA granted accelerated approval to Novartis's Gleevec (imatinib mesylate) for the treatment of patients with chronic myelogenous leukemia, which is largely seen as a success of the program.[21] The FDA's accelerated approval pathway led to significant controversy in 2021, however, when it was used to approve Biogen/Eisai's Aduhelm (aducanumab) for Alzheimer's disease.[22] As part of the swift backlash from this decision, several experts published an op-ed article in the *New England Journal of Medicine*, noting that "the FDA's decision is at odds with the evidence and with the agency's biostatistical review. The overwhelming unmet need in this common and devastating disease should drive research investments, not [a] lowering of regulatory standards that Americans rely on for safe and effective medicines."[23] The controversy has led the Office of Inspector General in the US Department of Health & Human Services to review the accelerated approval pathway, based on "concerns due to alleged scientific disputes within the FDA, the advisory committee's vote against approval, allegations of an inappropriately close relationship between the FDA and the industry, and the FDA's use of the accelerated approval pathway."[24]

≡ The Prescription Drug User Fee Act (PDUFA) "authorizes [the] FDA to collect fees from companies that produce certain human drug and biological products. Since the passage of PDUFA, user fees have played an important role in expediting the drug approval process."[25] In light of the ongoing debates on the drug approval process, it is important to understand that the legislative authority for the PDUFA requires a reassessment every five years, in order to continually adjust it, with the goal of improving regulations in the approval process. In PDUFA II (1997), the 12-month standard review time was reduced to 10 months, and norms for scheduling meetings and more review guidance were given. PDUFA III (2002) included three years of support for postapproval and postmarket safety activities. It also developed provisions for good review management practices and inaugurated rolling applications were introduced.

In PDUFA IV (2007), risk evaluation and mitigation strategies, commonly referred to as REMS, were introduced. These were intended to help improve postmarket drug safety. PDUFA V was part of the Food and Drug Administration Safety and Innovation Act (FDASIA), signed into law on July 9, 2012. FDASIA created a "breakthrough therapy designation" that is meant to further expedite the development and review of new drugs that may offer a substantial improvement over available therapies for patients with serious or life-threatening diseases.[26] PDUFA VI, approved in 2017, included several adjustments to the user fee structure to account for inflation and the FDA's increased workload.[27] With the upcoming PDUFA VII deadline in 2022, it will be intriguing to see how the impact of COVID-19 and the controversy surrounding approval of Aduhelm (aducanumab) for Alzheimer's disease will be taken into consideration.

The regulatory process in the United States, as it stands today, allows the FDA to approve a drug if it provides benefits that outweigh its known and potential risks for the intended population. The structured framework in which the drug approval process takes place includes an analysis of the target condition and available treatments for it; an assessment of the benefits and risks, derived from clinical data; and strategies for managing risks. In the next chapter, I explore the path each medical breakthrough took, from clinical trials to regulatory filing.

chapter 8
The Path to Approval

According to the FDA's website, "advisory committees provide FDA with independent advice from outside experts on issues related to human and veterinary drugs, vaccines and other biological products, medical devices, and food. In general, advisory committees include a chair, several members, plus a consumer, industry, and sometimes a patient representative. Additional experts with special knowledge may be added for individual committee meetings as needed. Although the committees provide advice to the agency, FDA makes the final decisions."[1] On the surface, this explanation seems straightforward, and it is largely encompassed by the definition. Advisory committees, or AdComs, can also elicit a form of suspense, due to the layout and feel of the meeting.

At least 48 hours before the event is to occur, meeting materials are published on the FDA's website. These include both the submitting company's analysis of the clinical and preclinical trial data they have produced and an independent review by the FDA.[2]

The details of these documents can range from agreeing with the company's analysis and recommending a positive benefit-risk profile for the drug, or completely disagreeing with the analysis and requesting several additional studies that may need to be completed prior to approval. Then, at the AdCom meeting, the committee spends several hours discussing the data and the analyses by both the submitting company and the FDA.

Now the meetings are largely virtual, but prior to the COVID pandemic, they occurred in a large conference room at the FDA, with a U-shaped table for the committee members, a rope barrier separating them from the audience, and several cameras at the back of the room, filming the deliberations. During in-person meetings, a single projection screen was set up at the front, where PowerPoint presentations were shown to the committee. The meetings—even the current virtual ones—could also include a public forum, where patients, doctors, and other members of the medical community sign up to speak about their experiences with the relevant disease, in what can sometimes become heart-wrenching testimony.

Meetings conclude with a vote on the questions that have been put forth to the committee by the FDA. These votes can be extremely tense in certain circumstances, particularly when the FDA and the sponsoring company disagree in their analyses of the data. While the FDA's definition of AdComs notes that the agency makes the final decisions, negative votes certainly do not inspire confidence in potential approval for the product. (Such a situation added to the controversy in the approval of Aduhelm, a drug for the treatment of Alzheimer's disease, noted in chapter 7, as the AdCom vote was overwhelmingly negative).

≡ On July 12, 2017, the Oncologic Drugs Advisory Committee for Kymriah (also referred to as tisagenlecleucel, the CAR-T therapy that was effective in treating Emily Whitehead and others) was held at the FDA's White Oak Campus in Silver Spring, Maryland.[3] Carl June was in attendance, and Stephen Grupp spoke as part of Novartis's presentation of the collected data. The primary efficacy analysis in the clinical trial that supported the product was based on 63 subjects, with an overall response rate—that is, the percentage of patients who have a partial or complete response to therapy—in 52 subjects (82.5 percent). The safety analysis showed severe cytokine release syndrome (a systematic inflammatory response) in 32 out of 68 subjects (47 percent). The FDA convened the AdCom to seek opinions on potential post-marketing considerations for side effects, including cytokine release syndrome; a long-term follow-up study on the potential for secondary malignancies; and whether the benefits of this therapy would justify the risks if it was approved.

Tom Whitehead was the fourth speaker during afternoon session of the open public hearing regarding the cell therapy that had saved his daughter Emily's life. He began his testimony that afternoon by saying, "Hello. My name is Tom Whitehead. . . . It is an honor to share with you today how my daughter, Emily Whitehead, became the first child to be treated and cured of leukemia in the CTL019 [Kymriah] trial at the Children's Hospital of Philadelphia." He then proceeded to tell the amazing story of how Emily fared under the medical care of Steven Grupp when treated with Carl June's CAR-T product.

> "CTL019 [Kymriah] killed Emily's resistant leukemia in
> just 23 days and did what standard treatment couldn't do.
> It saved our daughter's life. This treatment has kept our
> family whole. . . . There are parents all over the world
> watching, waiting to hear that this treatment will be
> available to try before their child dies from cancer. We
> believe that when this treatment is approved, it will save
> thousands of children's lives around the world. I hope that
> someday all of you on this advisory committee can tell

your families for generations that you were part of the process that ended the use of toxic treatments like chemotherapy and radiation as standard treatment and turn[ed] blood cancers into a treatable disease that even after relapse, most people survive. . . . If you want to see what a cure looks like for relapsed ALL, she's standing right beside me, and it's because of this treatment. I would like to take this time to thank, personally thank, everyone that worked so hard for so many years to turn [out] this treatment and have it ready for Emily when she needed it. There are amazing people working on this very hard and missing a lot of times with their own families."

A discussion and then a vote by AdCom members followed Tom's testimony. One question they were asked to addressed was, "Considering the efficacy and safety results of Study B2202 [the pivotal clinical trial], is the benefit-risk profile of tisagenlecleucel [Kymriah] favorable for treatment of pediatric and young adult patients (age 3–25 years) with relapsed (second or later relapse) or refractory (failed to achieve remission to initial induction or reinduction chemotherapy) B-cell precursor acute lymphoblastic leukemia (ALL)?" The vote was a unanimous "Yes" (10 to 0). Several of the committee members stated that the product indeed addressed an unmet medical need in the ALL population, the responses to treatment with it were impressive, and the clinical data was of high quality. "I think this is most exciting thing I've seen in my lifetime," said Tim Cripe, an oncologist with Nationwide Children's Hospital in Columbus, Ohio.[4]

Carl June was named to *Time* magazine's annual list of the "100 Most Influential People" in 2018. Emily—12 years old at that point, cancer free, and cofounder (with Tom and Kari) of the nonprofit Emily Whitehead Foundation to raise awareness and research funds for childhood cancer—penned a statement about him:[5]

I was a fun and energetic child. Then I spent two years in a hospital getting cancer treatment, but it wasn't working for me. That's when my parents and I learned about an experimental treatment, called T cell, that would train my immune system to fight my cancer; it hadn't been tried on a pediatric patient before. My parents believed that this was the right choice for me, and we transferred to the Children's Hospital of Philadelphia to enter the trial.

After getting the treatment, I went into a 14-day coma and awakened on my seventh birthday. But the treatment had worked! We later learned that Dr. Carl June's research had created this treatment. Dr. June saved my life and had a huge impact on my family. Without him, I wouldn't be here today writing this—and my parents and I wouldn't be helping other kids beat cancer.

Dr. June is my hero! He saved my family.

On August 30, 2017, the FDA announced a "historic action" in approving Novartis's Kymriah for certain pediatric and young adult patients with a form of ALL.[6] The federal agency touted it as "the first gene therapy available in the United States, ushering in a new approach to the treatment of cancer and other serious and life-threatening diseases." Scientists, physicians, and patients around the world cheered this historic approval. Even Novartis's competitors, Kite Pharma and Juno Therapeutics, applauded the decision. "Today is not about business or competition," Arie Belldegrun, Kite's CEO, wrote in a blog before the AdCom vote. "Today, we [Kite and Novartis] are not rivals. Today is about advancing an exciting technology that has the potential to transform cancer treatment."[4]

Kite enrolled additional patients in an open-label pivotal clinical trial, called ZUMA-1 (named after Zuma Beach, California), seeking to obtain FDA approval for their T cell therapy after initial treatment successes with it, similar to Emily Dumler's journey. The product was now called KTE-C19, or axicabtagene ciloleucel (axi-cel for short). At the 2015 American Society of Hematology's annual meeting in December, the company had presented their results of the ZUMA-1 study for the first time, with an overall dataset generally consistent with the National Cancer Institute's data.

In September 2016, Kite once again reported positive results from an interim analysis of the ZUMA-1 trial.[7] Its objective response rate in the aggressive non-Hodgkin's lymphoma population was 76 percent, with 47 percent of them in complete remission. Belldegrun commented, "What started at the NCI over a decade ago with the pioneering work of Steven A. Rosenberg, M.D., Ph.D., has evolved into a technology that has the potential to fundamentally change the outlook of patients with cancer."

The final results of the ZUMA-1 trial, which formed the basis of Kite's biologics license application (BLA) to the FDA for approval to market Yescarta (axi-cel), included 101 treated patients with a median age of 58 years, and three median numbers from prior therapies. The overall response rate to axi-cel was 72 percent (73 subjects), with a median response time of less than one month (0.9 months).[8] Belldegrun recalls, "Seeing patients alive at the NCI was one thing, but to see data coming out of Texas, Boston, Florida, and to take them all together, you suddenly see the common thread. All of these patients in the hands of different physicians, having the same results." The robust responses from a larger group of patients confirmed that CAR-T could provide life-changing outcomes for patients with DLBCL, just like it did for Emily Dumler.

As Belldegrun realized, however, there were several one-off results in clinical research labs across the United States, but nobody believed that this type of therapy could be commercialized for broader use. "This is not something you can plan for because there had never been a company in the space before. There was no expert in commercialization of CAR-T therapy. Cindy [Butitta, the company's CFO] and I knew we would have to blaze yet another trail. The question was when." Kite and Belldegrun had the foresight to invest in manufacturing capacity, in the form of a 43,500-square-foot plant in El Segundo, California, in close proximity to Los Angeles International Airport. The plant's location was strategic, as it would expedite the receipt and shipment of engineered T cell therapies from and to patients across the United States and Europe. In biotechnology, exemplary results and careful execution, such as those exhibited by Kite, have the potential to pique the interest of larger biotechnology companies, which may then pursue various business opportunities, including collaborations, licensing agreements, or even the acquisition of the smaller company.

☰ Every year for the past 36 years, the J.P. Morgan Healthcare Conference in early January brings together almost all major industry stakeholders in what can only be described as a sea of corporate suits, pantsuits, and dresses in the streets of downtown San Francisco. Dr. Robert Urban, the global head of Johnson & Johnson Innovation puts it, the conference's purpose is "to reflect on the trajectory of the biotechnology industry and now healthcare in general. To see how we, as a community, can bring forward new medical advances that are needed all across the world."[9]

The first conference occurred in 1983 and was hosted by Hambrecht & Quist, which was acquired by Chase Manhattan Bank in 2000. Chase was subsequently acquired by the J.P. Morgan Company in 2001.[10] While the conference itself is held in the Westin St. Francis Hotel in San Francisco and has drawn speakers such as J.P. Morgan CEO Jamie Dimon, Bill Gates, and Joe Biden (when he was vice president) in recent history, the surrounding areas become networking hotspots where you're likely to find CEOs of major corporations, top investors, and venture capitalists, as well as entrepreneurs looking to break into the fray. Hotel rooms in such places as The Donatello, the Kimpton Sir Francis Drake Hotel, The Clift, The Marker, and Park Central become corporate boardrooms where meetings take place that will shape the industry for the coming year. After-hours networking ranges from cocktail hours to dinners, where rubbing shoulders with someone can potentially lead to a business relationship down the line.

In January 2017, rain came pouring down on the city during the conference, accompanied by gusty winds, which left the streets littered with inverted umbrellas and hotel lobbies filled with soaked clothes and squeaky shoes. Andrew Dickinson, senior vice president of corporate development at Gilead Sciences, a very successful $90 billion (at the time) biotechnology company based in Foster City, California, met informally with Helen Kim, executive vice president of business development at Kite, to discuss Gilead's interest in oncology.[11]

At that point, Gilead had overseen one of the best product launches of all time with Harvoni, a 12-week treatment for hepatitis C that has cure rates of more than 90 percent. Gilead's hepatitis C franchise yielded a revenue of approximately $12.5 billion to the company in 2015, but the amount had declined since then, due to the available pool of treatable patients having been cured, leading some to even question if curing patients may not be a "sustainable business model."[12] The declining revenue from the product had put Gilead in a situation where its shareholders were looking for the next product, or platform, to provide growth.

After this initial meeting, a confidentiality agreement was put into place on February 2017, "providing for the sharing of information with a purpose of discussing, evaluating, negotiating, and potentially entering into a business transaction."[11] Following this agreement, representatives from both Gilead and Kite met in

March, April, and May 2017 to discuss updates on clinical studies, manufacturing capabilities, other clinical programs, and general thoughts on partnerships and oncology. In late May 2017, John Milligan, president and CEO of Gilead, contacted Arie Belldegrun and requested a meeting to talk about recent interactions between the companies. In summer 2017, Milligan and Belldegrun spoke on several occasions, including conversations about several potential acquisition offers, which increased in value as the two companies negotiated on a price.

On August 28, 2017, Gilead Sciences and Kite Pharma announced that they had entered into a definitive agreement in which Gilead would acquire Kite for approximately $11.9 billion.[13] As Milligan stated in a press release, "We are greatly impressed with the Kite team and what they have accomplished and share their belief that cell therapy will be the cornerstone of treating cancer. Our similar cultures and histories of driving rapid innovation in order to bring more effective and safer products to as many patients as possible make this an excellent strategic fit." Belldegrun was also quoted: "From the release of our pivotal data for axi-cel, to our potential approval by the FDA, this is a year of milestones. Each and every accomplishment is a reflection of the talent that is unique to Kite. We are excited that Gilead, one of the most innovative companies in the industry, recognized this value and shares our passion for developing cutting-edge and potentially curative therapies for patients."

Furthermore, both CEOs highlighted the innovative nature of cell therapies, and CAR-T in particular. Milligan stated, "The field of cell therapy has advanced very quickly, to the point where the science and technology have opened a clear path toward a potential cure for patients." Belldegrun noted, "CAR-T has the potential to become one of the most powerful anti-cancer agents for hematologic cancers. With Gilead's expertise and support, we hope to fulfill that potential by rapidly accelerating our robust pipeline and next-generation research and manufacturing technologies for the benefit of patients around the world." The dollar value of this acquisition immediately gained traction with major media outlets, while the worth of these therapies and what they were able to do for patients was beginning to be understood outside the medical community.

On October 18, 2017, axi-cel (now called Yescarta) received FDA approval to treat adult patients with certain types of large B-cell lymphoma. "The FDA approval of Yescarta is a landmark for patients with relapsed or refractory large B-cell lymphoma. This approval would not have been possible without the courageous commitment of patients and clinicians, as well as the ongoing dedication of Kite's employees," said Belldegrun. "We must also recognize the FDA for their ability to embrace and support transformational new technologies that treat life-threatening illnesses. We believe this is only the beginning for CAR T therapies."[14]

From an entrepreneurial perspective, Belldegrun had taken another step forward in creating value for shareholders of the company. In an analysis conducted by Bruce Booth, a partner at Atlas Ventures, with Gilead's acquisition of Kite, the investors in the initial round of funding had a 114-times increase their original investment, and others who later bought into the company at the initial public offering (IPO) gained an 11-times return.[15]

≡ Juno Therapeutics' CAR-T candidate, called JCAR015, was being developed to treat relapsed or refractory B-cell acute lymphoblastic leukemia (ALL). It was enrolled a clinical trial named ROCKET. Unfortunately, on July 8, 2016, three patients died from cerebral edema (brain swelling cause by the presence of excessive fluid), leading the FDA to place the trial on a clinical hold.[16] (A clinical hold is "an order issued by FDA to the sponsor of a new drug application to delay a proposed clinical investigation or to suspend an ongoing investigation.")

A clinical hold order may apply to one or more of the investigations covered by an IND (investigational new drug application).[17] When a *proposed* study is placed on clinical hold, subjects are not given the investigational drug. When an *ongoing* study is placed on clinical hold, in the interest of patient safety, no new subjects are recruited, and patients already in the study should be taken off therapy involving the investigational drug, unless specifically permitted to continue by the FDA. The clinical hold was lifted in near-record time on July 12, 2016, when Juno said they would continue the trial without using fludarabine and instead only employ the chemotherapeutic drug cyclophosphamide.[18]

On November 23, 2016, the FDA placed another clinical hold on the ROCKET study, after two additional patients developed cerebral edema and died.[19] Nonetheless, the study had been showing the treatment's effectiveness, with a 77 percent complete response rate (the absence of all detectable cancer once a treatment is completed) and a 90 percent response in those with minimal ALL. Juno's CEO, Hans Bishop, noted that the company was at a crossroad with JCAR015: "We are faced with a difficult decision, considering the encouraging early efficacy data in this trial and the poor prognosis of these relapsed/refractory ALL patients, who have few, if any, treatment options."

At the time, it was believed that these issues could occur in all patients treated with CAR-T therapies (although we now know this is not the case), and some doctors were speculating that cerebral edema might have been due to the specific product or the patient population, rather than the strategy itself. As an article in *Science* magazine stated, "they're [the doctors] mostly in the dark and hope that additional research, including new animal models, could help explain what happened and why."[20]

For all their potential benefits, clinical trials and the development of new drugs are not without risks. Along with the success stories, there are also unforeseen circumstances that lead to loss.

A 24-year-old clinical trial participant in the ROCKET study, Max Vokhgelt, was the first to die of cerebral edema. His father, Michael Vokhgelt, stated, "I believe in the promise of CAR-T therapy, but if traditional tests don't always predict deadly toxicities, drug sponsors must be allowed to use more predictive tests that better predict what happens to clinical trial participants. It is FDA's responsibility to protect human health and safeguard the public from dangerous drugs. Shouldn't all available tests to predict safety be used? I don't want another family to go through what my family went through."[21] In March 2017, Juno Therapeutics stopped further development of JCAR015, with CEO Hans Bishop stating, "We have decided not to move forward with the ROCKET trial for JCAR015 at this time."[22]

In November 2017, at the Society for Immunotherapy of Cancer (SITC) annual meeting in Oxon Hill, Maryland, Juno scientists presented their internal analysis of what happened in the ROCKET trial and came up with a multitude of variables that may have led to the five deaths.[23] An inward look at what went wrong was, and will continue to be, an important exercise within the biotechnology industry, in order to truly achieve the best possible framework for developing life-changing medicines. The following issues were raised in Juno's analysis:

- the degree of disease burden (the effects of the disease on an individual),
- the variability of the individual patient's own T cells,
- the extremely rapid multiplication of the modified immune cells in the patients who died (6–8 days postinfusion, rather than 12–14 days), which may have led to additional neurotoxicity, and
- a breakdown in the patients' blood-brain barrier, and a higher baseline level of interleukin-15 (IL-15), another T cell growth factor.

The company identified three lessons learned from advancing a new product, JCAR017, into clinical development: (1) define the composition of the T cells, (2) develop a deeper understanding of the clinical factors associated with risk, and (3) use better pre-clinical models to predict risk.[24] In 2018, JCAR017, the company's next-generation CAR-T, showed an objective response rate of 75 percent with a six-month complete response rate of 34 percent in its clinical study (known as the TRANSCEND trial). On February 5, 2021, JCAR017 would be named Breyanzi after it received approval for treatment in adults with relapsed or refractory large-B-cell lymphoma, joining Kymriah and Yescarta.[25]

The JCAR017 study yielded results that piqued the interest of another large biotechnology company, Celgene Corporation, based in Summit, New Jersey. In 2015, Juno and Celgene established an initial 10-year collaboration agreement, where Celgene bought an equity stake in Juno, the smaller of the two companies.[26] On September 14, 2017, Juno's board of directors held a meeting and discussed the acquisition of Kite Pharma by Gilead. Juno's management had also held discussions with another publicly traded health care company about a potential collaboration on another CAR-T product being developed for the treatment of multiple myeloma. Both Juno and Celgene, as well as Juno and the other party, continued their dialogue for the remainder of 2017, with the other company (identified only as "Party A") eventually withdrawing their interest.

On January 22, 2018, Juno and Celgene issued a join press release announcing that Celgene would acquire Juno for approximately $9 billion.[27] Mark Alles, the CEO of Celgene at the time, said, "The acquisition of Juno builds on our shared vision to discover and develop transformative medicines for patients with incurable blood cancers. . . . Juno's advanced cellular immunotherapy portfolio and research capabilities strengthen Celgene's global leadership in hematology and adds new drivers for growth beyond 2020." Hans Bishop, Juno's president and CEO, noted that "the people at Juno channel their passion for science and patients towards a common goal of finding cures by creating cell therapies that help people live longer, better lives. . . . Continuing this work will take scientific prowess, manufacturing excellence and global reach. This union will provide all three."

In an analysis of Juno Therapeutics, the venture capital funding for the company was critical, as well as lucrative. As Bruce Booth noted, "That's a $1B win for ARCH [Venture Partners]."[15] Bob Nelsen's vision, as a managing partner at ARCH (see chapter 2), helped fundamentally transform cancer therapy, and it also netted an estimated 22-times return on a roughly $45 million investment.

≡ Spark Therapeutics, led by Jeff Marrazzo and Katherine High, was able to advance the first AAV gene therapy into a regulatory filing with the FDA after completing a clinical trial that was able to show benefits in patients with a form of vision impairment associated with an *RPE65* mutation.[28] The clinical trial used a test established at the Children's Hospital of Pennsylvania, called the multi-luminance mobility test (MLMT), that was designed to measure changes in functional vision—in other words, the ability to navigate through a maze at different light levels, ranging from a brightly lit office to a moonless summer night.

The FDA convened an advisory committee to discuss the merits of the product (voretigene neparvovec), as it did with Kymriah. One of the voting questions for the committee to look at was, "Considering the efficacy and safety information provided in the briefing document, as well as the presentations and discussions during the AC meeting, does voretigene neparvovec have an overall favorable benefit-risk profile for the treatment of patients with vision loss due to confirmed biallelic *RPE65* mutation–associated retinal dystrophy?"[29]

The public hearing section of the meeting included several patients who discussed the life-changing benefits of voretigene neparvovec.[30] For example, one patient in the clinical trial noted her experiences before and after therapy:

> Without this trial, I have no idea where I would be today. I remember 6 years ago my doctor told me that by the time I was 18 years old, I would be almost or completely blind. That's scary for anyone to imagine. A year passed, and I found myself struggling to go to school or anywhere that I shall wander. I found myself reading Braille and walking with a cane. My biggest dream was to be normal, to be like everyone else.... After having the surgery ... we removed the patch, and I remember opening my eye to the bright, colorful world. Before surgery, my vision was dark. It was like sunglasses over your eyes while looking through this little tunnel. I remember looking at my stuffed animal for the first time. I did not know you could see hairlines. I remember seeing my mom's face for the first time. One of the best things I have ever seen after surgery was the stars. I never knew that they were little dots that twinkled. However, I honestly say that rainbows are overrated by far.

With several stories such as this, the vote, like that for Kymriah, was a unanimous "Yes" (16 to 0).

On December 19, 2017, the FDA approved voretigene neparvovec (Luxturna) as "the first directly administered gene therapy approved in the U.S. to target a disease caused by mutations in a specific gene."[31] FDA Commissioner Scott Gottlieb noted that the approval "marks another first in the field of gene therapy—both in how the therapy works and in expanding the use of gene therapy beyond the treatment of cancer to the treatment of vision loss— and this milestone reinforces the potential of this breakthrough approach in treating a wide-range of challenging diseases.... I believe gene therapy will become a mainstay in treating, and maybe curing, many of our most devastating and intractable illnesses."

In March 2018, Jack Hogan, a 13-year-old with vision loss as a result of an *RPE65* gene mutation became the first commercial patient treated with Luxturna.[32] Prior to treatment, he was night-blind, and he most likely would become legally blind in his 20s or 30s. Two months later, "Jack can now see in light that is six times dimmer, and he can read fine print that is 40 percent smaller."[33] His surgeon, Jason Comander, noted, "These results are representative of just how big a moment this is for gene therapy. It is helping our patients, and it is here to stay."

≡ At the 2017 American Academy of Neurology (AAN) conference, Jerry Mendell delivered a presentation on results from the Phase I trial for AVXS-101 gene therapy, administered to 15 infants with spinal muscular atrophy type 1 (SMA1).[34] The data showed dramatic improvements in motor skills in most of the babies, with all of the patients remaining alive and none of them requiring ventilation at 13.6 months, an age at which 75 percent of untreated infants have either died or require ventilation. Additionally, eight patients could sit up unassisted, and two could crawl, stand, or walk independently—a milestone that is usually never seen in SMA 1 babies. The highlight of Mendell's presentation was a video of Matteo Almeida (see chapter 4) walking down a hallway to an elevator, carrying an electronic toy, and then reaching up to press a button, a feat that drew a standing ovation from the audience and emotional responses from nurses and caregivers who were in attendance. Mendell noted that Matteo was "basically completely back to normal. You see and examine him; it just about takes your breath away."

The results presented at the AAN conference were an interim analysis of the study, and a data cutoff at a later date was published in the *New England Journal of Medicine*.[35] As of August 7, 2017, all 15 patients were alive and no longer needed assisted ventilation at 20 months of age, compared with an 8 percent rate of survival in one study of the natural history of the disease. Further, of the 12 patients who received the dose that AveXis now planned to use for a pivotal trial, "11 sat unassisted, 9 rolled over, 11 fed orally and could speak, and 2 walked independently."

This study, as well as a Phase III study for Spinraza, a drug to treat children and adults with SMA2, were highlighted in NIH director Francis Collins's blog: "What if, rather than tricking cells into producing SMN protein [with Spinraza], it were possible to simply correct the genetic defect that's responsible for SMA in the first place, by supplying a functioning copy of the responsible gene? It might sound too good to be true, but the second paper in the *New England Journal of Medicine* [Mendell et al.'s AVXS-101 results] reports results from this exact strategy. And, while longer-term study is needed, the results are again extremely encouraging."[36]

Similar to the stories of drug developments by Kite Pharma and Juno Therapeutics, the clinical benefits for patients and the innovation that AVXS-101 represented caught the eye of larger biotechnology companies. In this case, AveXis had been contacted be several suitors as early as 2015.[37] In December 2017, after the November publication of the AVXS-101 study's results and the company's announcement that the FDA had permitted them to initiate a pivotal trial in SMA type 1 patients, as well as a trial in SMA type 2 patients using an intrathecal route of administration (i.e., through the spinal canal), Charles Bailey, Novartis's head of business development and licensing for neuroscience, contacted R. A. Session II, AveXis's senior vice president for corporate strategy and business development, to make an introduction and potentially get together at the upcoming J.P. Morgan Healthcare Conference.

While the representatives were unable to meet, the companies remained in contact throughout early 2018, with several negotiations over an acquisition price taking place. On April 9, 2018, Novartis announced the company's intent to acquire AveXis for $8.9 billion. In the company's press release, the CEO of Novartis, Vas Narasimhan, stated, "The proposed acquisition of AveXis offers an extraordinary opportunity to transform the care of SMA. We believe AVXS-101 could create a lifetime of possibilities for the children and families impacted by this devastating condition."[38] AveXis had now joined Kite Pharma and Juno Therapeutics as multibillion-dollar acquisitions in the cell and gene therapy field, all within a roughly nine-month span. On May 24, 2019, Zolgensma (AVXS-101's commercial name) was "approved for the treatment of pediatric patients less than 2 years of age with spinal muscular atrophy."[39]

≡ In February 2014, the FDA held a public meeting for sickle cell disease patients to hear perspectives on the most significant effects of their disease and available therapies.[44] Several key themes were identified, including the following:

1. The health effects of sickle cell disease were wide-ranging (episodic pain crises, acute chest syndrome, and chronic fatigue and cognitive effects).
2. The disease takes an emotional toll.
3. Currently approved therapies have significant intrapatient variability.
4. There is a need for better treatments.

The FDA took the feedback from this meeting and published a report discussing a benefit-risk assessment framework, concluding that "the current treatment options are effective in reducing the number and severity of sickle cell disease complications. However, their efficacy varies from patient to patient, and significant treatment burden and side effects can limit benefits or preclude use of treatment." Furthermore, the feedback noted that "the disease remains suboptimally managed in a significant portion of the population."

The National Institutes of Health has an ongoing Cure Sickle Cell initiative, to "take advantage of the latest genetic discoveries and technological advances to move the most promising genetic-based curative therapies safely into clinical trials."[46] Progress in this area has even led some regulatory officials to opine that we might see cures for diseases like sickle cell anemia within 10 years. Currently, sickle cell anemia remains an unmet medical need, with a patient population that is looking to be treated equitably.

These initiatives, and the advancements made to date, provide hope that the disease will be tamed by *ex vivo* gene therapy. As Alexis Thompson, at the Ann and Robert H. Lurie Children's Hospital in Chicago, sums up, "The Cure Sickle Cell Initiative is a bold and visionary plan to bring potential cures to the broader community of individuals living with SCD. The fact that the National Institutes of Health has taken on this important challenge sends a powerful message to individuals with SCD and their health care providers that moving promising science from the laboratory bench to the clinic is a real priority for the United States government."[47]

Sickle cell disease affects a worldwide population, where global delivery and access will be important. A working group called the Global Gene Therapy Initiative (GGTI) was formed to "tackle the barriers to low-and middle-income countries inclusion in gene therapy development" by engaging key stakeholders to find coherent and pragmatic solutions . . . so that, without exception, patients in need can have access to gene therapy no matter where they reside."[48] Additionally, a recent article describing efforts by the Bill & Melinda Gates Foundation and the Novartis Institutes for BioMedical Research notes that specific needs in resource-limited areas of the world include single-administration "shot-in-the-arm" gene therapy interventions, local health systems that are able to diagnose patients and ensure their well-being until the treatment can be administered, and the development of financial and delivery models to make gene therapies accessible to all.[49] The authors note that "a functional 'cure' of sickle cell anemia by *in vivo* gene therapy would historically transform the clinical management of the disease while also potentially generating technology platforms that could be applicable to *in vivo* gene therapies for other diseases, including HIV."

There is a clear need for effective and tolerable treatment options for patients to improve their daily functioning and reduce long-term complications. *Ex vivo* gene therapies are being developed by several companies—including but not limited to, bluebird bio and CRISPR Therapeutics/Vertex—with the goal of curing sickle cell disease.[45] These have not yet been approved by regulatory authorities but are showing signs that they may provide a major advancement in therapeutic options. These therapies, barring any unforeseen safety issues that develop over time, most likely will be headed for potential regulatory approvals.

part II

Enabling the Next Wave of Innovation

chapter 9
Building Blocks

n the first part of this book I explored three examples of medical breakthroughs:

1. CAR-T therapy for the treatment of leukemia and lymphoma in patients such as Emily Whitehead and Emily Dumler, leading to three FDA approved products: Kymriah, Yescarta, and Breyanzi (chapter 2).
2. *In vivo* gene therapy using AAV in spinal muscular atrophy, which treated patients such as Matteo Almeida and led to the FDA approved product Zolgensma (chapter 4), as well as to Luxturna in cases of vision loss related to a *RPE65* gene mutation (chapter 8).
3. *Ex vivo* gene therapy in sickle cell anemia, a significant unmet medical need that impacts patients such as Terry Jackson, is showing robust benefits in treated patients like Victoria Gray (chapter 6).

While each situation is unique, in my view, there were key building blocks in place for these breakthroughs that can also be applied to create the next wave.

Perseverance

Scientific breakthroughs are built on the foundation of decades of research. Both cell and gene therapies fall directly into this niche. The path to the development of the first three FDA approved products involved almost five decades of research since the concept was first proposed.[1] Furthermore, the serious adverse events in this field led to a reexamination of the basic science, in order to create safer products. Perhaps an inflection point, or "Eureka" moment, may involve some aspect of luck. Nonetheless, it is built on years, sometimes decades, and even centuries of incremental discoveries that can be attributed to persistence.

In Adam Grant's *Originals: How Non-Conformists Change the World*, he challenges the myth of glorified entrepreneurs as ultimate risk-takers—the ones who go all-in on a venture without any regard for the risks—and instead shows that they are driven less by risk and more by the opportunity to try something new.[2] "To become original, you have to try something new, which means accepting some measure of risk," Grant writes. "But the most successful originals are not the daredevils who leap before they look. They are the ones who reluctantly tiptoe to the edge of a cliff, calculate the rate of descent, triple-check their parachutes, and set up a safety net at the bottom just in case." This couldn't be truer for the majority of biotechnology entrepreneurs, as both the basic science and the proof-of-concept research must be completed prior to starting a company and securing millions of dollars and funding. Perseverance remains a key factor in determining the trajectory of a breakthrough in medicine.

Never Stop Learning

The most improbable part of Carl June's story with CAR-T therapy was his ability to identify an elevated level of the protein IL-6 in Emily Whitehead and suggest using tocilizumab, based on his understanding of the breakthroughs occurring in the treatment of rheumatoid arthritis. Jerry Mendell took the lessons learned and the success of the AVXS-101 clinical trials for spinal muscular atrophy and is putting them to use in order to develop additional gene therapies with the potential to treat other neuromuscular diseases, such as Duchenne muscular dystrophy and limb-girdle muscular dystrophy.

Gene therapies for sickle cell disease continue to drive improvements in cell manufacturing techniques, in order to create potentially better products. In Walter Isaacson's biography of Leonardo Da Vinci, he encourages readers to "observe" and "go down rabbit holes," based on lessons from the life of one of the most outstanding minds ever known.[3] As he emphasizes, "Leonardo's greatest skill was his acute ability to observe things.... He drilled down for the pure joy of geeking out." Breakthroughs in medicine will only be generated by the collective push to explore the unknown and take risks, yet they will mainly rely on society to create incentives for broad-scale intellectual curiosity.

Embrace and Learn from Failure

The need to destigmatize failure is correlated with continually learning. In a Nike commercial, Michael Jordan famously says, "I've missed more than nine thousand shots in my career. I've lost almost three hundred games. Twenty-six times, I've been trusted to take the game-winning shot and missed. I've failed over and over again, and that is why I succeed." This same approach to taking risks needs to be applied and reinforced in relation to both basic science and drug development.

With sophisticated computational tools, reductions in the time necessary to conduct proof-of-concept experiments, and a greater understanding of basic human biology, we are already trending toward more favorable outcomes early on in the clinical trial process by identifying red flags sooner. For example, realizing a model system has a drug-related toxicity, and either shelving a potential compound or altering it slightly to overcome its negative effects, are steps that increasingly take place in the developmental stages of products.

Nonetheless, in a *Harvard Business Review* article coauthored by Noubar Afeyan, the founder of Flagship Pioneering (the company from which Moderna emerged) and Gary Pisano, they believe it is important to create an environment where programs die as a result of being less competitive with other programs, a type of Darwinian evolution (or what Afeyan calls "emergent discovery"), versus the glorification of a decision to kill a program.[4] Further, "in striving for breakthrough innovation, the predominant strategy today is the 'shots on goal' approach—the antithesis of emergent discovery. It entails funding a large portfolio of projects in the hope that the profits from the rare success will more than pay for the cost of the numerous failures. . . . But the shots-on-goal approach ignores the fact that breakthrough concepts are usually riddled with flaws at the outset. . . . Because the mantra of the shots-on-goal approach is to kill early and often, many promising ideas struggle to survive past the embryonic phase."

On an individual level, research suggests that we're afraid to take risks because we emphasize the potential negative outcomes, and "losses loom larger than gains" in the decision-making process.[5] Psychology research delineates a common four-step cycle we go through in response to bad outcomes: attention, reaction, explanation, and adaptation.[6]

First, there's a recognition of failure and our response to it, which commonly involves a negative emotion (fear, surprise, anger, etc.). The explanation process occurs when we begin to understand what happened. This is where research shows that a distinction can occur between how we view our own failure versus that of others. In other words, do we consider it simply bad luck or some inexplicable difficulty, rather than our own fault, when evaluating ourselves but do the opposite when looking at what happens to others?[7] Adaptation is where we have the opportunity to gather new information from a lack of success. As a society, learning from failure and destigmatizing it will be a key step toward continued innovation.

Be Willing to Change Course

Innovation includes the ability to boldly change course when facts do not support an underlying hypothesis. Biology, chemistry, and physics are tools with which we attempt to understand the world around us, but sometimes the laws of nature are counterintuitive and don't fit into a simple story. Innovation is dependent on the ability of leaders in the field to efficiently adapt to changing environments. For example, when the Human Genome Project was initiated, determining the genetic blueprint of a human being seemed to be a simply way of unveiling the drivers of disease. The end result did not have that type of immediate impact, and we learned that the body's way of packaging, processing, and expressing information was quite a bit more complicated.

This understanding played a role in investments in several other areas of research, such as epigenetics—namely, the study of inherited modifications in genes that do not involve changes in the underlying DNA sequence. Overall, a reduction in the costs of gene sequencing, an ability to collect and analyze big data, and groundbreaking work from the race to encode human DNA continues to be part of the foundation for our understanding of disease, but maybe not in the way it was first imagined.

Build an Environment that Promotes Thinking "Outside the Box"

Incentivizing curative therapies; bringing in new stakeholders (such as private foundations) or new government initiatives (like "All of Us") to increase the open sourcing of data sets; and encouraging collaboration across disciplines will help build and maintain an environment that will produce breakthroughs in medicine. In *The Tipping Point—How Little Things Can Make a Big Difference*, Malcolm Gladwell notes, "If you want to bring a fundamental change in people's belief and behavior . . . you need to create a community around them, where those new beliefs can be practiced and expressed and nurtured."[8] In order to solve some of the most pressing challenges in health care, investing in and nurturing talent must remain a key focus.

Two publications examining the age at which Nobel laureates conducted their prize-winning work show that achievements in medicine generally occur at a later point, compared with those in more theoretical fields, such as physics, potentially due to the training requirements and experimental work conducted across one's life cycle of the field of medicine.[9,10] Therefore, particularly in science, investing in talented individuals at an early stage in their careers and maintaining adequate funding for their work may be paramount to their ability to make a breakthrough in their respective fields.

Another study explored the origins of 252 new drugs that were approved by the FDA from 1998 to 2007.[11] It also defined whether the drugs were scientifically innovative and responded to unmet medical needs, as well as assessed the relative contributions of pharmaceutical companies, biotechnology firms, and universities to those products. The analysis suggested that biotechnology companies, and universities that transferred their discoveries to such firms, accounted for roughly half of the FDA-approved drugs that were scientifically innovative, as well as half of the drugs that responded to unmet medical needs. Factors that were considered in assessing why the United States outperformed other countries included public funding for academic biomedical research, the peer review process in allotting grants, career flexibility for biomedical researchers (along with favorable social attitudes toward switching jobs and being employed in the private sector), and a supportive culture of entrepreneurship in the biotechnology industry.

Lastly, a paper from the University of Chicago and Northwestern University examined 65 million journal articles, patents, and software products produced from 1954 to 2014, in order to determine how the character of science and technology differed when produced by large teams versus small teams.[12] For each dataset, the authors assessed the degree of disruption in each subgroup (articles, patents, and software products) and found that it was substantially greater in work by small teams than that by large groups. Progress from larger teams was built on developments that were more recent and popular, with their results gaining attention sooner. The authors concluded that "both small and large teams are essential to a flourishing ecology of science and technology" and suggested that "to achieve this, science policies should aim to support a diversity of team sizes."

Each of these publications describe factors that are critical for the maintenance of an environment that encourages bold new approaches to the development of medicines to treat diseases.

Collaboration and the Importance of Social Capital

Steve Jobs, in his product-launch presentations, famously showed a slide of the intersection between "Liberal Arts" and "Technology" Streets as the inspirational source for Apple's creativity and innovation. We are now arriving at the intersection of "Health Care" and "Technology" Streets, where embracing the knowledge gained from each discipline and leveraging expertise can promote exponential growth in several areas. While stories of lone wolf scientists or entrepreneurs gain notoriety, some of the largest global initiatives were what laid the foundation for many of our current breakthroughs in medicine. Continued work at the crossroad of the knowledge economy's two most innovative sectors must be encouraged if we are to achieve the ambitious goal of curing disease.

While many of the inflection points are built on a consensus of scientific truths and studies from laboratories that arose from either previous work or an understanding of foundational concepts, the idea of social capital is critical in each of this book's stories of scientists and entrepreneurs. Social capital is defined as a concept that involves the potential of individuals to secure benefits and invent solutions to problems through their membership in social networks. The definition includes three dimensions:[13]

1. interconnected networks of relationships between individuals and groups,
2. levels of trust that characterize these ties, and
3. resources and benefits that are both gained and transferred by virtue of social ties and social participation.

In the three examples I have discussed (as well as in the epilogue, when I will cover breakthroughs associated with COVID-19), there were key scientific and business relationships, developed over the course of careers, that allowed these breakthroughs to flourish. The right place and the right time are crucial, but the right people with the right expertise are also required.

Competition

In each of the breakthroughs I've discussed, there is an underlying current of true competition between groups, which is integral to this process. With scientific discoveries, a focus on solving a particular problem or answering a specific question can result in additional datasets, which than have the potential to spawn multiple other problems and questions. Maintaining a focus on being the first to build and then disseminate news of a breakthrough does not occur as efficiently without competitive forces driving it. Moreover, as coronavirus research during the COVID-19 pandemic has shown, competition does not need to inhibit collaboration. In scientific research, probably more than in any other field, collaboration and competition, working in harmony, may be integral in creating breakthroughs.

Incentivization

The importance of incentivization—that is, something that arouses action or activity—and the allocation of resources remain key factors in building breakthroughs. One important facet is the fact that large amounts of investment in biotechnology occur at the preclinical and pre-revenue parts of the process, several years prior to a therapeutic treatment reaching the subsequent stages of clinical trials, regulatory filing, and approval. Therefore, the value of these companies is based on projections of future revenues. The more impactful the drug, the higher its potential use in patients with the relevant disease. This alignment leads to reinvestments in talent and promising scientific ideas, and, often, the subsequent formation of a new company. I further explore the importance of different types of incentivization and investment in chapters 10 and 11, but these two mechanisms that drive innovation are critical to building breakthroughs.

The Big Idea

The above themes are certainly not new. Nonetheless, they are pervasive throughout this book's stories of recent breakthroughs. Gene and cell therapies have worked their way through various challenges and iterations to get where they are today, with champions shepherding these ideas through to their realization as therapeutic products. My examples have shown the breakthrough moments in the lives of some of the initial patients treated with these therapies and highlighted the effectiveness of these developments when employed in larger studies of severe diseases.

From my perspective, the next wave of innovation will not be as technologically constrained and thus may favor strategies built around big, bold ideas. President Kennedy's original moonshot proposal was both inspiring and tangible. It was also able to galvanize a nation by creating the space race. Beau Biden's "Cancer Moonshot" idea (to find a cure for cancer) and the Chan-Zuckerberg Initiative's goal of curing, preventing, and managing all disease by the end of the century are similarly ambitious. Operation Warp Speed was able to advance therapeutic and vaccine progress exponentially during the COVID-19 pandemic, compared with standard development times.

Therefore, can we be on the cusp of truly pursuing "moonshot" ideas in biotechnology? Large datasets have now been generated, which can truly begin applying artificial intelligence and machine-learning platforms to identify targets for therapeutic intervention, as well as potentially enhancing our ability to recognize and prevent diseases from occurring (or, at least, to identify them at an earlier stage in their progression). We now have technologies that are capable of editing any "letter" of the DNA code in a genome. In addition, synthetic biology, a multidisciplinary area of research that has the potential to either create new biological systems or redesign ones already found in nature, is a burgeoning field.

≡ With the advent of these complex medical treatments, which are part procedure and part therapeutic, questions will invariably arise. How do we use an accelerated approval system to balance the need for critical analysis and a desire to quickly use a treatment? How do we adequately value the benefits of novel therapies, approved for one-time use, within the structures of our medical reimbursement system? And how do we continue to nurture the growth and scaling up of these breakthroughs? In the next chapter, I discuss attributes that could enable the next wave of innovation, which include medical reimbursement models, continued investment in new therapies, incentives to pursue breakthroughs, and means of developing talent.

chapter 10
Recognizing Value

In discussing drug development, it is almost impossible to avoid the elephant in the room—pricing. Opinions on potential legislative changes regarding drug prices (there are sure to be several on this topic alone) are not within the scope of this book, but arguments have been made for the need to create payment models that account for the disruptive value of certain products.

The fervor around the topic of drug prices picked up substantially on a chilly February afternoon in 2016, when Martin Shkreli sat in the US House of Representatives and said, "I intend to follow the advice of my counsel, not yours. . . . I evoke my Fifth Amendment privilege against self-incrimination and respectfully decline to answer your question."[1] His black hair had probably been combed for the first time in several months and gave the appearance of somebody taking this event seriously, but his facial stubble was in sharp contrast to this neat hairstyle and reflected an attitude of disdain and indifference. That year, Shkreli, the CEO of Turing Pharmaceuticals, had become the face of the pharmaceutical industry to the general public.

The FDA approved Daraprim (pyrimethamine), used in combination with leucovorin, to treat toxoplasmosis, which can be a life-threatening parasitic infection in patients with weakened immune systems (such as individuals who have AIDS, are on chemotherapy, or have received an organ transplant). Shkreli's initial notoriety, which earned him the nickname "Pharma Bro," came from acquiring the rights to Daraprim and raising its price from $13.50 a pill to $750 a pill, an increase of over 5,000 percent. This business model of taking advantage of the inelastic pricing environment in the pharmaceutical industry, as well as of a small patient population impacted by a life-threatening disease, was seen by most as a demonstration of greed. Public outrage from the sticker shock of Daraprim's new cost highlighted an issue that was boiling for several years and finally spilled over into the general consciousness.

During a hearing in the House of Representatives, one congressman after another used quotations from Shkreli's previous interviews in an attempt to get him to respond to their questions and comments. First up was the chairman of the committee, Jason Chaffetz of Utah: "What do you say to that sick old pregnant woman who might have AIDS, no income, she needs Daraprim to survive, what do you say to her?" Shkreli responded by merely invoking his Fifth Amendment rights.

Then Congressman Trey Gowdy of South Carolina noted, "You gave an interview to a television station in New York, if I understood you correctly, where you couldn't wait to come educate the members of Congress on drug pricing." Shkreli again took the Fifth. That was his reply once more when Congressman Elijah Cummings of Maryland implored, "I want to plead with you to use any remaining influence you have over your former company to press them to lower the price of the drug. . . . You can look away if you like, but I wish you can see the faces of people that cannot get drugs that they need. . . . Somebody's paying for these drugs, it's the taxpayers that are paying for some of them."

After an uneventful eight-minute exchange, it became clear the Shkreli had no intention of answering any questions, and he was dismissed from the hearing. With the light of major media coverage shining brightly on Shkreli for those few weeks, much of the general public found him to be particularly repulsive. For example, in January 2017, GQ magazine dubbed him the "most hated millennial in America."[2]

In an email sent to the chairman of the board of Turing Pharmaceuticals regarding the company's progress in acquiring Daraprim, Shkreli stated, "$1 b[illio]n here we come."[3] Later, in an email to an outside contact, he highlighted, "We raised the price from $1,700 per bottle to $75,000. . . . So 5,000 paying bottles at the new price is $375,000,000—almost all of it is profit and I think we will get 3 years of that or more." Political rhetoric from both sides of the aisle on the increasing cost of drugs has consistently found a sounding board in the public.

≡ A plethora of news stories are bringing attention to the growing problem of rising health care costs in the United States, including drug pricing. For example, an article in the *Washington Post* described a patient diagnosed at age 13 with Ewing sarcoma, a type of cancer that occurs in the bones or the soft tissue around them, mainly affecting children and young adults.[4] She was treated with an aggressive regimen of radiation and chemotherapy and later developed breast and thyroid cancer, as well as heart and lung problems. Even with health insurance, her out-of-pocket costs were approximately $12,000 a year for medical care and prescription drugs, a substantial financial burden for the average household.

Another article in the *New York Times* discussed several such cases.[5] One was that of a 57-year-old woman from Minneapolis with an income of less than $20,000 who couldn't afford the 12 prescribed medications for her congestive heart failure, diabetes, and related complications. Another was the situation of a 24-year-old man from Oakland, California, who was diagnosed with chronic myelogenous leukemia (cancer of the white blood cells) and was prescribed Gleevec, which required him to dip into his student loans for law school.

Most of us can empathize with the real-time financial hardships people face in order to receive needed medical care. The issue has grown to the point where even the National Cancer Institute has given it a name, financial toxicity.[6] This refers to "problems a patient has related to the cost of medical care. Not having health insurance or having a lot of costs for medical care not covered by health insurance can cause financial problems and may lead to debt and bankruptcy. Financial toxicity can also affect a patient's quality of life and access to medical care. For example, a patient may not take a prescription medicine or may avoid going to the doctor to save money." According to a study by the Kaiser Family Foundation, in 2019, Americans filled an average of 11.6 prescriptions per year, a trend that is likely to continue to grow with an aging population.[7]

The issue is particularly striking in terms of cancer. Such patients are more likely to incur financial toxicity than people without this disease, since older patients are at greater risk for developing cancer. A study conducted at St. Jude's Hospital analyzed 2,811 long-term survivors who faced financial hardships, as measured by three different endpoints.[8] It found that 22.4 percent, 51.1 percent, and 33 percent of the participants reported material, psychological, and coping/behavioral hardships, respectively.

Patients should have access to effective treatments. Additionally, the pursuit of innovation should persist in producing breakthrough therapies to further improve patients' health, the health care system in general, and society. If this occurs, new and better medicines will continue to transform the treatment of devastating diseases.

≡ Total spending on retail prescription drugs has remained flat (when accounting for inflation), at 12 percent, with net brand-name drug prices falling for the past four consecutive years.[9,10] One study examined the relative prices of generic and branded, or brand-name, drugs from 2008 to 2014 and showed that the number of manufacturers for a generic drug was strongly associated with its relative price. For drugs with only one generic manufacturer, their cost to patients was 87 percent of that for the brand-name version. For drugs with a second generic manufacturer, this decreased to 77 percent. Three generic manufacturers dropped the relative price still further, to 60 percent, and the average decline increased with having even more manufacturers.[11] Therefore, if a drug initially cost $100, its price would be $87 with one competitor, $77 with a second competitor, $60 with three competitors, and so on, all the way down to $21 with ten or more competitors.

The hepatitis C market is a case study of innovation in biotechnology and cost savings arising with competition, despite it being initially lumped into the outrage over Martin Shkreli and Daraprim.[12] Prior to the recent wave of new therapies, the treatment for hepatitis C involved injections of the drug interferon. This procedure often came with flulike symptoms, lasted six months to a year, and only cured approximately 40 to 50 percent of the patients. Additionally, patients with advanced liver disease couldn't receive these injections. Under this treatment regimen, data from the Centers for Disease Control suggested that more than 60 percent of people with hepatitis C would end up with chronic liver disease, and as many as 20 percent would develop cirrhosis of the liver. A liver transplant, the only option for some at this point, would cost roughly $600,000.[13]

In December 2013, Gilead Sciences' Sovaldi (sofosbuvir) was approved for the treatment of chronic hepatitis C as a once-daily oral drug.[14] As Ira Jacobsen, chief of the Division of Gastroenterology and Hepatology at Weill Cornell Medical College, noted, "Sovaldi will have a major impact on public health by significantly increasing the number of Americans who are cured of hepatitis C." Sovaldi, in combination with other agents, achieved very high cure rates (in the 90 percent range), in addition to shortening the duration of the treatment to as little as 12 weeks and reducing or completely eliminating the need for interferon injections.

This breakthrough was followed in October 2014 by the approval of Gilead's Harvoni (a combination of ledipasvir and sofosbuvir), the first once-daily, single-tablet regimen for chronic hepatitis C that shortened the treatment period to weeks for some patients. While its initial price was thought to be too high by some,[15] the drug not only represented a medical breakthrough after years of research, but it was also more curative and safer than the previous standard of care. It also saved the health care system from the potential costs related to chronic liver disease, cirrhosis, and liver transplants. Within a few years of Harvoni's commercialization, competitive products entered the market and cut the cost per patient by more than 60 percent over the price of the first entrant.

In 2017, Peter Bach at the Memorial Sloan Kettering Cancer Center and Mark Trushiem at MIT's Center for Biomedical Innovation made a financial case that the US government should buy Gilead Sciences on the open market for $156 billion: "Buying the company rather than purchasing its products just works out to be a far cheaper route."[16] The authors claimed that by looking at other factors that could sweeten the deal, "at a final net cost of around $32B the government can provide free drug to all others, including veterans and active military, federal and state employees, prisoners, and those in Medicare and Medicaid." In 2019, the state of Louisiana proposed a "Netflix-like" subscription model, where the state would pay a fee to a drug company to get unlimited access to the drug, "with the goal of treating 10,000 hepatitis C patients in its Medicaid and prison population."[17]

Placing a premium on innovation creates an incentive for the development of breakthrough medicines. The key for maintaining biotechnology's social contract to provide innovative therapies is to renew confidence in the life cycle of developments shifting from brand name to generic drugs.[18]

One idea that gained traction in the biotechnology industry was to institute a type of Hippocratic oath for companies. The Hippocratic oath, in its original Greek form, required a new physician to swear on the healing gods to uphold professional ethical standards. The Declaration of Geneva, a modernization of this oath, was adopted by the World Medical Association in 1948 and most recently revised in 2017.[19] The oath asks members of the medical profession to pledge their dedication to the health and well-being of their patients, using good medical practices, without employing demographic considerations.

Understanding and conveying the importance of developing medicines to society, as well as regaining trust, is of the utmost urgency for the biotechnology industry. In a viewpoint published in *Nature*, Bob More, a member of the venture capital firm Alta Partners, notes, "When we [as an industry] see practices that put profits ahead of patient needs, we need to call foul publicly and not look the other away. We need to move away from gimmicks that raise only the price of drugs, not their value. People who use these tricks should be fired. Their projects should be shunned by venture capitalists and potential funding partners. . . . If the pharmaceutical industry is to thrive, we must all embrace the Hippocratic oath, whether in academia, business, finance or at the bench. The cost of lost trust to the drug industry is worth much more than manipulated short-term gains."[20]

An article in the *Harvard Business Review* discusses four tactics that drug developers use in an attempt to stop the entry of generic drugs and arrest the cycle leading from branded to generic forms:[21]

1. "Pay for delay" agreements, where a branded drug company pays a generic firm not to launch a version of a drug. The Federal Trade Commission estimates that this practice cost the United States $3.5 billion per year.
2. A "citizen petition," which asks the FDA to delay action on a pending generic application. In a review of this program, the FDA noted that branded drug manufacturers filed approximately 92 percent of the so-called citizen's petitions between 2008 and 2015.
3. The creation of "authorized generics," which "aren't really generic products at all; they are the same product sold under a generic name by the company that sells the branded drug. Why? By law, the first generic company to market a drug gets an exclusivity period of 180 days. During this time, no other companies can market a generic product."
4. The original drug developer restricts the use of brand-name samples to testing purposes only, by declining to sell them on the open market.

Arguably, ending some of these tactics is a way to increase transparency in the life cycle of drug marketing and rebuild trust in the genericization of branded products. This would make way for a new wave of transformative therapies—an iterative process of innovation that rewards the proper parties for altering the course of medical afflictions in society.

The benefits to the global community from medical breakthroughs over the past half century have been staggering. Life expectancy in the United States has increased substantially over the past 40 years. Worldwide, life expectancy has doubled in some areas. The field of *curative* therapies—which cell and gene therapies may eventually represent—will, if successfully implemented, inherently reduce the population of patients that require treatment, as has been shown for hepatitis C. In what Merck, a multinational pharmaceutical company, calls "a defining moment," in 1950 its founder, George W. Merck, said, 'We try to remember that medicine is for the patient. We try never to forget that medicine is for the people. It is not for the profits. The profits follow, and if we have remembered that, they have never failed to appear. The better we have remembered it, the larger they have been."[22] Creating a model where biotechnology companies no longer have an incentive to discover and develop cures for diseases would be detrimental to innovation. Additionally, renewed trust in the competitive life cycle of brand-name to generic drugs, or biologic to biosimilar drugs, needs to be established for a currently skeptical public.

☰ A key issue impacting the drug-pricing debate is a fee-for-service structure in which doctors and health care providers are paid for each service performed. This is particularly true for cell and gene therapies. They are transformative but extremely complex and, therefore, have a very expensive price tag. Despite the innovative nature of these therapies, sticker shock remains a concern among the public, as exemplified by an article in the *Wall Street Journal* that discusses the list prices for Kymriah ($475,000) and Yescarta ($373,000).[23]

The creation of either new or alternative financing models for health care under the heading of value-based payment arrangements is important in encouraging the development of breakthroughs in medicine and potentially curative therapies. The fee-for-service model, as a driver of the increased costs of health care, has been a major point of contention among experts as the total amount of health care spending in the United States continues to grow.[24]

So where did fee-for-service come from? In the early twentieth century, various states proposed compulsory health insurance, but all the proposals failed. From the 1920s to 1930s, the demographics of the US population shifted, and the scientific era began. In *The Care of Strangers: The Rise of America's Hospital System*, Charles Rosenberg notes, "By the 1920s . . . prospective patients were influenced not only by the hope of healing, but by the image of a new kind of medicine—precise, scientific and effective."[25] From the late 1920s through the 1960s, the concept of health insurance grew. In 1929, Blue Cross Plans were established "to provide pre-paid hospital care based on a prototype developed by Baylor University in Dallas, Texas," where a group of school teachers contracted with Baylor Hospital to provide up to 21 days of hospitalization for $6 per year.[26]

The fee-for-service payment model worked well for much of the twentieth century, because most patient problems were acute in nature—that is, new, rather than long term (chronic). In that context, fee-for-service allowed easy access to affordable medical care and rewarded doctors appropriately. Over the past 30 years, however, the complexity of patient conditions and medical treatments has changed dramatically, whereas the reimbursement system has not. As more people began to experience chronic diseases, and the available treatments grew in both number and expense, problems from excess utilization began to outweigh the benefits of this system.[24]

The term "value-based payment" has gained popularity in many health care circles in recent years, as an alternative to the fee-for-service model. At its core, value-based payment is intended to align pricing with the expected benefits from outcomes in a particular therapy. Changing the health care system from payments for a service—such as buying a cup of coffee—to a model where prices are based on the value of a therapy's transformative benefit will incentivize cures. Determining what should be considered "value" and how it should be defined remains an important point in this debate.

≡ Value-based payment arrangements were first used in the 1990s, when Merck guaranteed payment refunds for cholesterol-lowering drugs that did not help patients meet target levels. Since then, the appetite for these types of contracts continues to grow, particularly in an age of personalized medicine, with electronic medical records providing better measures of patient results and "real world" evidence. A 2017 report by McKinsey and company estimated that Italy had been the leader in the development of publicly disclosed value-based contracts since 1994, with 73, although The United States was second, with 49.[27] European markets also "largely led the development of innovative arrangements in the 1990s."

Another article analyzed several case studies of value-based payment arrangements from 2003 to 2008, which included drugs such as Novartis's Lucentis (for the treatment of wet age-related macular degeneration) and Merck's Januvia/Janumet (for diabetes).[28] Lucentis is administered as an injection into the eye once a month for three months, to help a patient's diminishing eyesight. If that patient loses a specified amount of vision, another injection in necessary.[29] A 2008 arrangement included Novartis limiting reimbursements to the United Kingdom's National Health Services to 14 injections, after which the company would pay for the product directly.[30] The agreement required Novartis to maintain a registry on each patient and their visual acuity, and to reimburse a hospital for any doses beyond that limit.

In 2009, Merck and Cigna (a pharmacy benefits management company) entered into the first US outcomes-based pharmacy contract agreement for Merck's diabetes medications, Januvia and Janumet.[31,32] Merck would provide discounts to Cigna when people with type 2 diabetes who were in Cigna's diabetes support program were able to lower their blood sugar levels, regardless of the medication they were taking. Merck would further increase the rebate if the patients who were prescribed Merck's drugs (Januvia or Janumet) took their medications according to their physicians' instructions. This arrangement between Merck and Cigna increased the percentage for enrollees with type 2 diabetes who were able to control their blood sugar levels by taking Januvia or Janumet appropriately, with savings of as much as $8,000 per patient.

Between 2015 and 2017, 16 risk-sharing contracts were publicly announced, more than double the number in the previous two decades.[33] For payers and providers, these types of contracts could mitigate risk and address a product's performance in the real world, compared with a clinical trial. For manufacturers, value-based payment arrangements could help with market penetration and differentiation if their product is truly innovative and provides substantial benefits over the current standard of care.

White papers for the Duke-Margolis Center for Health Policy's Value-Based Payment Consortium—composed of academics, biotech/pharmaceutical company members, pharmacy-benefit managers, and health care insurers—discuss two types of payment contracts.[34,35] Indication-based contracts have the goal of pricing a drug according to its use in treating a particular disease, following evidence generated in its risk-benefit profile. Outcome-based contracts link payment for medical products to their actual performance in a patient or group of patients.

As part of a broader effort to develop value-based payment frameworks, the advisory group identified several current obstacles to the increased use of these arrangements in the United States. These include the infrastructure for and constraints on real-time data collection and difficulties in implementing payment contracts, as well as the federal government's anti-kickback statute, government pricing challenges, and the FDA's regulation of communications between payers and manufacturers.

Novartis's Kymriah and Spark Therapeutics' Luxturna were introduced as having a potential for rebates, based on both their effectiveness and other pilot program reimbursement measures. These first-in-class drug development companies intended to show that they were serious about furthering the promise of value-based payment frameworks.

Kymriah offered an outcome-based approach, where payment for the drug would be made only when pediatric and young adult ALL patients respond by the end of the first month.[36] A cost-benefit analysis on Kymriah (and Yescarta) concluded that these CAR-T therapies "seem to be priced in alignment with clinical benefits over a lifetime time horizon."[37] Spark Therapeutics developed three value-based payment arrangements for Luxturna:[38]

1. An outcome-based rebate program agreement with two private payers where, if the treatment failed in "both short-term efficacy (30–90 days) and longer-term durability (30 months)," Spark would return a portion of the $850,000 price tag for this one-time therapy.
2. A demonstration project with the Centers for Medicare & Medicaid Services that would enable Spark to offer private and governmental payers "an installment payment option, as well as greater rebates to clinical outcomes."
3. A patient access program that would reduce the financial risk and burden for payers and treatment centers by entering into an agreement where the payer would agree to provide coverage for its members, Spark would assume all in-transit, storage, and handling risks for the drug, and the payer and treatment center would separately agree on reimbursement for the specialized medical care required to deliver the product.

In August 2018, the Alliance for Regenerative Medicine Foundation for Cell and Gene Medicine released an analysis that sought to establish several additional inputs to measure in a value-based reimbursement framework: patient population size, a lifetime horizon of value, indirect costs (i.e., costs associated with a loss of productivity), nonmedical costs for patients and caregivers (both during treatment and over a patient's lifetime), a patient's age at the onset of the disease, additional value for curative therapies, real-world evidence, societal economic impact, and patient-centered endpoints.[39]

An analysis of the value-based pricing of Novartis's Zolgensma estimated it to be $1.1 to $2.1 million per patient.[40] Novartis subsequently priced Zolgensma at $2.1 million, offering insurers the possibility of paying annual installments of $425,000 over the course of five years.[41] Another example is bluebird bio's LentiGlobin, which was developed for the treatment of transfusion-dependent beta thalassemia. In January 2019, the company calculated this drug's "intrinsic value" to patients at $2.1 million.[42] In June of that year, bluebird bio said that in Europe, it would price Zynteglo (the commercial name for LentiGlobin) at €1.575 million ($1.77 million) for the total treatment, but offered a "five-year, results-driven installment payment plan."[43] After an initial payment of €315,000, patients would be charged the same amount per year for the remaining four years only if the one-time therapy provided benefits for them.

Overall, the intent of these models is to further the eventual goal of value-based payment arrangements—that is, increasing the push for innovation in biotechnology discovery, and focusing on development to produce better outcomes for patients. An article by authors from the pharmaceutical industry and from the Duke-Margolis Center for Health Policy noted, "Now is a particularly opportune time to develop value-based payment arrangements for gene therapies. The short-term per-patient costs of one-time, curative treatments may be relatively high—leading to more pressure to demonstrate value in practice, including value over time. . . . Fine-tuning these approaches to support potentially high-value gene therapies is a critical and urgent part of achieving an innovative and affordable health care system that is truly focused on curing and preventing diseases."[44]

Given this push for innovation, combined with the seemingly endless debate on pricing, the question is where we, as a society, should place our resources to achieve these results. A 2021 letter from biotechnology industry executives to President Biden and congressional leaders notes, "We are concerned about the high and rising out-of-pocket costs that have made our medicines increasingly unaffordable to many patients. . . . To solve the problem of affordability for patients, we must lower the amount that insurance plans can make patients pay out-of-pocket, redefining proper insurance by law, just as policymakers have appropriately outlawed discrimination on the basis of pre-existing conditions."[45]

The letter then continues, "Translating those ideas [basic research funded by the NIH] into actual medicines is almost entirely driven by the private sector and makes all that basic research worth funding in the first place. . . . The NIH and industry are parts of one whole ecosystem, not a replacement for one another. . . . Preserving market-based incentives for drug R&D [research and development] is how we get the medicines to achieve this goal."

So what does the current environment of early-stage drug development and investment look like? What are the areas in which we can improve our means of generating the next breakthrough in medicine? The next chapter examines how investors approach biotechnology venture capital, investments in basic science, and the need to nurture and motivate the next generation of scientists.

chapter 11
Financial and Human Capital Investments in Biotechnology

The age-old debate about the value of basic scientific research and its impact on society still exists, particularly in times of constrained resources, when it may be more practical to fund projects where a clear link from an idea to its outcome is established. One study, published in 2018, examined the importance of fundamental research to today's important drugs by analyzing 28 of the "most transformative" medicines approved for clinical use by the FDA between 1985 and 2009.[1] The authors determined that many of these "were made without regard to practical outcome and with their relevance to therapeutics only appearing decades later." Approximately 80 percent of the medicines examined were able to be linked with one or several basic discoveries.

Another study focused on the research and development costs of 68 randomly selected new drugs.[2] Both publications suggested that there was a 20-year incubation period (most likely taking place in academia) before formal projects began in pharmaceutical companies, due to the potential risks associated with product development. Subsequently, it takes about 10 to 12 years before a developer files a new drug application for the product with the FDA. Dr. George Yancopolous, the chief scientific officer of Regeneron Pharmaceuticals, when commenting on drug development, has said, "Quantitatively, it is the single hardest thing that we do as a society."[3]

The translation of concepts into therapies involves rigorous science, as well as an understanding of how to take discoveries and develop them into a commercially viable drug. While government funding has an important part in advancing the basic science, private investment is paramount in making innovative medicines. Here is where venture capitalists and entrepreneurs, particularly in the life sciences, play a vital role.

≡ In 1975, Robert ("Bob") Arthur Swanson, a 28-year-old venture capitalist, began cold calling prominent scientists in the field of recombinant DNA. This technology uses enzymes to cut and then paste together pieces of DNA that are of interest to researchers. The recombined DNA sequences can be placed into vehicles called vectors, which ferry the DNA into a suitable host cell, where it can be copied, or replicated, in bacteria or yeast.[4] According to *Genentech: The Beginnings of Biotech*, "Without exception, all believed recombinant DNA had industrial promise but surmised it would require a decade or two of development before commercial payoff."[5] Swanson remained persistent in his interest and eventually called Herb Boyer, a biochemistry professor at the University of California, San Francisco (UCSF). Boyer agreed to meet with Swenson for 10 minutes on a Friday afternoon.

The initial 10 minutes became three hours, and their office conversation then moved to a neighborhood tavern for "at least as many beers." The two started a company they called Genentech (Boyer's suggestion, and a much better name than Swanson's idea, "HerBob"). Their fateful meeting, considered by many to be the birth of the biotechnology industry, is encapsulated in a bronze statue that sits on Genentech's campus. In March 1976, Swanson presented a six-page preliminary business plan that the two had developed together to his former employer, Kleiner & Perkins, after being rebuffed by a scion of a California banking family. Genentech's stated mission was "to engage in the development of unique microorganisms that are capable of producing products that will significantly better mankind," as well as "to manufacture and market those products."

Swanson requested $500,000 in startup funds, but Kleiner & Perkins agreed to invest $100,000. By May 1978, Genentech had created two chains of insulin in bacteria, and on August 21, 1978, the first molecules of recombinant insulin were formed in a test tube. On October 14, 1980 Genentech issued 1.1 million shares of stock, at $35 a share, in its initial public offering (IPO).[6]

In pre-pandemic times, the IPO process involved a "road show," a one-to-two-week jaunt across the world with back-to-back investor meetings in different cities and countries, with the intent to sell large blocks of the company's proposed stock. As Fred Middleton, the third member of the founding team with Herb Boyer and Bob Swanson, recalls:[7]

> People just listened and gaped. Herb got up and did his
> trick with the pop beads, showing how recombinant DNA
> works. . . . Basically, we had a little clear plastic box with
> pop beads in it—the baby toys that pop together. [The box]
> was supposed to represent bacterium. He took out the
> beads and showed how you spliced genes together. . . . The
> fact that a UCSF professor was up there explaining it had
> everyone mesmerized. I gave the talk on the financial side,
> Bob gave the talk on the strategy, Herb gave the talk on
> the technology. . . . Every time we asked for questions
> there weren't any. People didn't know what to ask. There

were no experts, there were no analysts. Everybody was just amazed.

A minute after the opening bell on October 14, Genentech shares skyrocketed from $35 to $80, peaking at $89 within 20 minutes and settling for the day at $71. Based on the closing price, the company's value was estimated at $532 million. Boyer and Swanson, holding 925,000 shares apiece, earned approximately $70 million in a one-day profit. In 1990, Genentech and Roche announced a merger transaction where Roche would own 60 percent of the equity in Genentech, paying $2.1 billion.[8] In March 2009, Roche agreed to acquire full ownership of Genentech for $46.8 billion, ending "what is widely considered the world's oldest and most successful biotechnology company" at the time.[9]

Genentech's success spawned an industry that continues to grow, both in the size of financing for it and the number of investors. Investments in health care companies has doubled every two years since 2017, from $16 billion to $34 billion to more than $80 billion in 2021.[10] The key metric for venture capitalists to consider, however, is a return on invested capital, adding another layer of complexity to the push for biotechnology innovation.

≡ In the 2010 movie, *The Social Network*,[11] Mark Zuckerberg (played by Jesse Eisenberg, with curly, unkempt hair and dressed in a black North Face jacket and yellow shirt), and Sean Parker (played by Justin Timberlake, wearing a suit coat, white t-shirt, and glasses) meet with entrepreneur and venture capitalist Peter Thiel to secure funds for their start-up company. Thiel served as Facebook's "angel investor," providing a now-famous $500,000 in capital in exchange for 10.2 percent of the company. That initial investment has turned into well over $1 billion, with Thiel netting $640 million soon after the company completed their IPO in May 2012.[12] Moreover, Thiel's funds were not the only ones that generated outsized returns. Facebook also netted a potential 800-times return on a $12.7 million Series A investment for Accel Partners, in a deal that valued the company at $98 million.[13,14]

These types of returns have become legendary in Silicon Valley, joining such deals as the 350-times returns for Kleiner, Perkins, Caufield, and Byers (KPCB) and Sequoia Capital—now some of the most successful venture capital firms ever—for their investment in Google.[15] In 1999, KPCB and Sequoia each put $12.5 million into Google for a 10 percent stake, which was worth approximately $2 billion at Google's IPO. Other tech deals that have reached this level are now common names in day-to-day conversations, and some have even become verbs in and of themselves, such as "facebooking," "tweeting", and "ubering." As Bijan Salehizadeh and Bruce Booth, two life sciences venture capitalists, described in a 2011 *Nature Biotechnology* commentary, "Although life sciences investing creates new medicines . . . within the venture capital asset class it has often been treated like an ugly stepchild relative to its 'high tech' sisters focused on new software, Web 2.0, clean tech, and social media."[16]

To understand how venture capital investments in the life sciences compare with the more well-known ones in technology, an evaluation of returns across different venture capital sectors found that from 2000 to 2010, health care venture capital investing yielded a gross pooled mean invested rate of return of 15 percent for "realized deals" (i.e., deals where investors sold or otherwise disposed of their shares) and 7.4 percent for realized deals plus the value of the active unrealized investment.[17] These numbers were higher than those for all the technology venture sectors that were analyzed, such as hardware, software, and internet technologies, as well as the S&P 500's return over the decade.

Additionally, the overall failure rates (i.e., making less than or only equaling the initial investment) for life sciences occurred in 58 percent of the realized investments in this time horizon, versus 75 percent for technology investments. Excluding the year 2000 (notable for the burst of the "dot-com bubble"), loss rates in the life sciences dropped to 56 percent, and those in technology to 68 percent. These data also highlight the high risk–high reward nature of venture capital, regardless of the sector. On the success-rate side, over 8 percent of deals in the life sciences in the 2000s had a 5-times or greater return on investment, versus 4 percent of the technology deals. Whether this trend will continue is unknown. Nonetheless, the number of stakeholders interested in investing in the life sciences industry has grown considerably.

A goal for many venture capitalists is to achieve a 3-times gross rate of return on each fund.[18] Therefore, determining the appropriate fund size is key to calculating the amount needed to achieve these goals. The higher the amount of money raised, the greater the number of deals that will need to be generated at an acceptable rate of return on the initial investment.

Venture capital funding has grown since 1998, with a majority of the capital committed to investment funds of $300 million or more. With this trend, a term that has become more and more important in venture capital investment is "capital efficiency," where the greatest amount of value can be generated per dollar invested.[19] This has been thought to be a function of two major factors:

1. Capital intensity, or the total amount of equity investment required to create a value inflection point, such as an IPO or an acquisition.
2. The cost-of-capital, or the rate of return new investors will demand in order to invest.

Only capital intensity can truly be controlled, and it is dependent on several factors, including the amount of capital needed, how much money is necessary to work on the most important aspect of the proposed project, and timing. Moreover, does the investment come at an appropriate price?

Some of these same considerations can be exemplified by *Moneyball: The Art of Winning an Unfair Game* (later made into a movie starring Brad Pitt).[20] The book follows the 2003 Oakland Athletics baseball team and their general manager at the time, Billy Beane, focusing on his analytical and evidence-based approach to assembling a team: "In what amounted to a systematic scientific investigation of their sport, the Oakland front office had reexamined everything from the market price of foot speed to the inherent difference between the average major league player and the superior Triple-A one. That's how they found their bargains." While a life sciences venture capitalist has to take into account a different set of variables from the one that determines the success or failure of a baseball team, an important consideration that is consistent between the two is the ability to nurture and assess talent and fill roles appropriately, in order to increase the efficiency of the respective organizations.

Approximately 400–500 biopharmaceutical companies are financed every year, which is, surprisingly, consistent from year to year. Even with the greater influx of venture capital in recent years, the total number of companies has stayed relatively flat, making the average amount of venture capital per investment substantially higher.[21] So where's the bottleneck, if the resources exist?

As Bruce Booth says, "The big issue is a talent problem and the need for experienced talent that knows drug research and development . . . particularly, the integration of skills around the business of science is crucial, and a lot of those skills require time." Clearly, the infrastructure that supports the early and mid-career development of talented scientists, the environment of collaboration to achieve scientific breakthroughs, and the types of institutions that are involved all need to evolve to meet the increased speed of communications provided by technology. The good news is that there are several promising ideas that, if implemented, may help achieve the goals of enhancing the talent pipeline and streamlining the process that leads from lab-bench research to bedside treatment, in order to expedite the development of curative therapies.

≡ In early 2018, the proposed yearly budget for the National Institutes of Health was between \$34 billion and \$36 billion. In terms of purchasing power (and adjusted for inflation), that amount was down by roughly 20 percent from 2003.[22] That lack of growth in funding is decreasing the number of grant applications (with fewer discoveries being made) and reducing the number of young, talented researchers who receive funding (thus killing the talent pipeline).

A 2016 study examined the demographics among research project grantees awardees at the National Heart, Lung, and Blood Institute (NHLBI).[23] The analysis showed that since 1998, the proportion of established (ages 56 to 70 and older) investigators who received research project grants (RPGs) was increasing in a "slowly progressive and strikingly linear fashion," compared with 1998, when mid-career (ages 41–55) investigators constituted 60 percent of all researchers who received a grant. The remaining 40 percent was divided between early stage (ages 24–40) and established investigators. The study warned, "A collateral result of these demographic shifts, when combined with level or declining funding, is a significant reduction in the number of RPG awards received by NHLBI mid-career investigators and a corresponding decrease in the number of independent research laboratories."

Laurie Glimcher, president and CEO of the Dana-Farber Cancer Institute, corroborated this analysis at the 2017 Forbes Healthcare Conference: "They [academic medical centers] train the next generation of doctors. They do groundbreaking research that leads to new cures and they take care of very complicated patients, but they are under severe threat, squeezed by shrinking health care reimbursements in the face of increasing cost of healthcare and shrinking NIH budget."[24] Nonetheless, there are several steps that can be taken to enlarge the talent pipeline, encourage collaboration to generate improved outcomes, and expedite the lab-bench to bedside development of drugs.

This sentiment was echoed by Bill Gates at the 2018 J.P. Morgan Healthcare Conference, where he noted the importance of three sectors:[25]

1. Government-funded basic science, which "shines a light on promising pathways to health advances."
2. Philanthropy, which "can help nurture the best ideas through discovery and development, and balance the risk-reward equation for private-sector partners."
3. The life sciences industry, which "has the skills, experience, and capacity necessary to turn discoveries into commercially viable products."

Regarding government-funded science, innovative frameworks, developed with multiple stakeholders, to create large and diverse open source datasets that can be utilized freely continue to pay dividends. An example of this is the Cancer Genome Atlas (TCGA) collaboration between the National Cancer Institute and the National Human Genome Research Institute. TCGA has generated comprehensive multidimensional maps of the key genomic changes in 33 types of cancer and made them publicly available.[26]

The 21st Century Cures Act was signed into law by President Barack Obama on December 13, 2016.[27] On that occasion, he discussed the role of American innovation: "One of my highest priorities as President has been to unleash the full force of American innovation to some of the biggest challenges that we face. That meant restoring science to its rightful place. It meant funding the research and development that's always kept America on the cutting edge.... It meant investing in the medical breakthroughs that have the power to cure disease and help all of us live healthier, longer lives."[28] This act provided the FDA with new, expedited development programs, including the Regenerative Medicine Advanced Therapy program and the Breakthrough Devices program. The law also authorized $500 million in funding over nine years to help the FDA carry out provisions of the act, as well as to develop a work plan for their implementation.[29]

On July 25, 2018, Scott Gottlieb of the FDA testified before a US House of Representatives subcommittee on the ongoing implementation of the 21st Century Cures Act.[30] In addition to exploring potential data-sharing initiatives, the FDA was modernizing its internal framework to encourage collaboration across divisions where approaches had become more complex and interdisciplinary. For example, the FDA's new Oncology Center of Excellence began focusing on a specific disease area, rather than a type of product. This initiative later led to FDA approval, in May 2017, of Merck's Keytruda (pembrolizumab), the first cancer treatment based on aspects of a tumor's biomarkers, or genetic signature, rather than where the tumor was located, which is how most cancers are defined (think "lung" or "colon").[31] Gottlieb also described the FDA's efforts to encourage novel clinical trial designs, advance drug development tools, and integrate real-world evidence from electronic health records, registries, and claims and billing data, in order to improve our knowledge of diseases.

In an article in the *New England Journal of Medicine*, Francis Collins and Kathy Hudson, from the National Institutes of Health, commented on the impact of the 21st Century Cures Act in reducing "bureaucratic red tape," facilitating the exchange of data in a safe manner, and funding three "highly innovative scientific initiatives":[32]

1. The Beau Biden Cancer Moonshot, to double the rate of progress in the fight against cancer, make more therapies available to a larger number of patients, and improve the

medical field's ability to detect cancer, which received $1.8 billion in funding over 10 years.

2. The Brain Research through Advancing Innovative Neuro-technologies (BRAIN) Initiative, to build further knowledge in real-time brain function, which received $1.5 billion in funding over 10 years.

3. The Precision Medicine Initiative, to further advance health research in individualized prevention and treatment, which received $1.46 billion in funding over 10 years.

Philanthropic foundations are notably increasing their footprint in life sciences research. One of the oldest foundations, the Howard Hughes Medical Institute (HHMI), began in the late 1940s with a small group of physicians and scientists who advised aviator and industrialist Howard R. Hughes.[33] Hughes created the institute on December 17, 1953, with the intent of pursuing basic research and probing into "the genesis of life itself." According to the HHMI Charter, "The primary purpose and objective of this corporation shall be the promotion of human knowledge, . . . principally in fields associated with basic biomedical sciences, and the dissemination and application of that knowledge for the benefit of humanity." The institute has been wildly successful, with its flagship research effort, the HHMI Investigator Program, having collaborated with over 60 US institutions to provide support for more than 250 scientists and their research teams. More than 180 HHMI investigators are members of the National Academy of Sciences, and the institute has supported more than 30 Nobel laureates.[34]

The most well-known philanthropic effort is the Bill & Melinda Gates Foundation. It started in 1997, with the couple reading an article about millions of children in poor countries who died from diseases that were eliminated in the United States. The current entity was formed in 2002, when the William H. Gates

Foundation merged with the Gates Learning Foundation. In 2006, the foundation restructured its priorities to focus on three issues: global health, global development, and programs in the United States.[35,36] That year, Warren Buffet also pledging $30 billion for "improving the lives of millions of fellow humans who have not been as lucky as the three of us." The foundation is "guided by the belief that every life has equal value" and "works to help all people lead health, productive lives." Its investments have led to new drugs and vector control tools for malaria, accelerated the introduction of new vaccines, improved access to contraception, and expanded and simplified antiretroviral treatment for HIV.

The Gates foundation has also made investments in companies like Immunocore (using T-cell technology to help stimulate the body's immune system) and Moderna (using messenger RNA, or mRNA, for vaccine and drug development). In his speech at the 2018 J.P. Morgan Conference, Gates ended with a message to the biotech companies and investors who were in attendance, one that strikes to the core tenet of an innovative framework using collaborations between the foundation and industry: "Over the last decade, our experience has shown that we can stretch the reach of market forces so the private sector's most exciting innovations also benefit people with the most urgent needs. And with creative thinking, we can do it in ways that are both sustainable and profitable. Our foundation is in a unique position to share the risk on promising bets that can lead to important new discoveries. And we can help provide more predictability to companies interested in entering new markets that present real challenges, but also tremendous opportunities."[37]

Other frameworks for advancing science were also recently initiated by Sean Parker, as well as by Mark Zuckerberg and Priscilla Chan. Parker created the Parker Institute for Cancer Immunotherapy, in order to "accelerate the development of breakthrough immune therapies to turn cancer into a curable disease."[38] The initiative's approach is to encourage strategic partnerships and share tools, infrastructure, and data across their membership, including academia, nonprofit institutions, biotech, and pharma. A key focus of the institute is to advance T cell therapies, such as CAR-T, as well as the science surrounding drug resistance by some cancers, in order to find new targets to attack and create a greater understanding of the role immunotherapy can play in treating the disease.

The Chan-Zuckerberg Initiative (CZI) was launched on September 21, 2016 with a Facebook announcement and a goal of "supporting scientific research to help cure, prevent, and manage all diseases."[39] The CZI would focus on "bringing scientists and engineers together to build new tools that can empower the whole scientific community to make breakthroughs on the four major disease categories": heart disease, cancer, infectious disease, and neurological disease like stroke. The financial commitment from this initiative was $3 billion, spread over 10 years, including $600 million to fund a research center in San Francisco, called the BioHub, where scientific and medical researchers would work alongside engineers on long-term projects.[40]

In an article discussing the CZI and the broader importance of philanthropy in the sciences, Nobel laureate David Baltimore noted that Chan and Zuckerberg's announcement "joins forces with other philanthropists to push the envelope and support audacious ideas, with long-term commitments, to solve some of our greatest challenges."[41] He concluded by stating, "These gifts are certainly broadcasting a common message—philanthropists recognize that a long view of progress is worth investing in."

In December 2021, the Arc Institute, a new research institution for "curiosity-driven biomedical science and technology," was cofounded by Silvana Konermann, Patrick Hsu, and Patrick Collison.[42] Its mission is to accelerate scientific progress and understand the root causes of complex diseases. Influenced by the Howard

Hughes Medical Institute and the Chan-Zuckerberg Initiative, it will provide full "hard money" support (more than $650 million committed to scientists in eight-year renewable terms) for investigators, close partnerships with a number of major research universities, investments in technology, a long-term career path for researchers, and physical co-location for researchers. As Konermann explained, "It's not that the current model is really bad for everyone—I think the current model actually works really well for some people. . . . The hope is not that everything will be like Arc, but that each of these models will have their own downsides and their own upsides," making "a 'healthier ecosystem.'"[43]

By increasing and fortifying the talent pipeline with investments in basic scientific research, as well as giving innovative thinkers the ability to work on ambitious long-term challenges, encouraging new and current stakeholders to invest and collaborate using unique business models, and adequately rewarding the high-risk stakes of drug development, the environment for creating the next generation of breakthroughs in medicine will be maintained. In the next chapter, I touch on what this may be.

chapter 12
Looking Forward

The race to map the human genome, via the Human Genome Project (HGP), was one of the largest undertakings in science in the twenty-first century.[1] HGP provided the first draft of roughly 3 million base pairs that make up a human's DNA sequence. This began with a joint announcement in June 2000 and dual publications in 2001 from HGP (an international consortium) and J. Craig Venter's Celera Genomics, a for-profit company based in Rockville, Maryland.[2,3] Since that initial undertaking was completed, scientists would periodically update a "reference genome."

Roughly 8 percent was still missing from the most up-to-date reference genome until two scientists—Adam Phillippy, a computational biologist at the National Human Genome Research Institute, and Karen Miga, a geneticist at the University of California, Santa Cruz—founded the Telomere-to-Telomere Consortium in 2019 to complete the sequencing.[4] In 2021, the consortium published six papers, including "The Complete Sequence of a Human

Genome," which provided "the first complete 3.055 billion base pair sequence of a human genome, representing the largest improvement to the human reference genome since its initial release."[5]

Using this reference genome, a line of research called genome wide association studies, or GWAS, has shed light on how some diseases are linked to genetic variants, identifying more than 200,000 of them. Many initially assumed that GWAS and the sequencing of the human genome were going to lead to answers on more widespread diseases.

As a result of this work, it did become clear that the characteristics of the diverse genetic strains that are linked to human disease are highly variable. As an article in *Science* notes, "This architecture is the consequence of the interplay between demographic and selective forces from our species' evolutionary history."[6] Over the coming decade, examining deep whole-genome sequencing, in combination with functional data, will provide greater insight into novel mechanisms on how diseases are manifesting—that is, displaying characteristic signs or symptoms—which, in turn, may allow more targeted therapeutics to be developed.

The costs associated with diagnostic tools and genome sequencing continue to decrease, allowing the formation of companies that can collate huge datasets and provide further understanding of what factors determine the development and the degree of severity of diseases. To put the growth of DNA sequencing (and the resultant cost decrease) in perspective, the National Human Genome Research Institute (NHGRI) tracked the costs associated with DNA sequencing performed at centers funded by the institute.[7] It compared this data with Moore's Law, which states that overall processing power for computers will double every two years.[8]

What the NHGRI study found was that, beginning in January 2008, the cost per genome began to substantially outpace Moore's

Law, most likely due to the transition from a slower sequencing method (called Sanger sequencing) to next-generation DNA sequencing technologies that were exponentially reducing timelines.[9,10] The first human genome project took 13 years, and cost estimates range from $1 billion to $3.8 billion. In 2018, the Rady Children's Institute for Genomic Medicine set the Guinness World Record for the time needed to decode rare genetic disorders in newborns through DNA sequencing—19.5 hours—besting their prior 2015 record of 26 hours.[11] The cost of sequencing an entire genome is now below $1,000 per individual, with goals to reach $100 per individual.[12]

The intersection of progress in understanding human biology and the economic feasibility of generating and understanding large datasets presents a substantial opportunity to benefit society by creating newer, more targeted medicines to treat disease. Furthermore, the potential applications of artificial intelligence and machine-learning platforms to the large swaths of data already being generated are just starting to be explored. While the initial sequencing of the human genome provided the dictionary of how human beings are genetically encoded, we are now beginning to be able to speak that language and create smarter medicines, as well as more complex models to test them.

In addition to robust data generation and analysis, we are entering a renaissance era in biotechnology, where gene therapy, cell therapy, and gene-editing candidates have the goal of producing curative products that target the underlying etiology, or cause, of the disease. The clinical outcomes described earlier in this book are only scratching the surface of what's possible. Investments in next-generation therapies highlight the optimistic sentiment and enthusiasm generated by these treatments.

By the end of the third quarter of 2020, there were approximately 1026 regenerative medicine and advanced therapy companies worldwide, including 547 in North America, 244 in Europe and Israel, and 199 in Asia.[13] Furthermore, global financing for these companies in the first three-quarters of 2020 totaled $15.9 billion, an increase of 115 percent. Not only have early-stage venture capitalists participated in this process, but larger institutional investors and pharmaceutical companies have also committed significant amounts of capital. With public financing as the main driver—along with IPOs ($2.8 billion) and follow-on financing, also called supplemental funding ($5.7 billion)—the amount surpassed that of previous years.

Regulatory authorities worldwide have further solidified this capital influx by accepting these therapies, which create real benefits for society, and identifying what they view as redundancies in the review process. The Recombinant DNA Advisory Committee (RAC) was established in 1974 to advise NIH's director on research that used emerging technologies, including elements of genetic material.[14] The FDA began to regulate gene therapy products in 1984.[15,16]

Since this time, efforts to understand the basic biology of disease and the differential methods for delivering gene therapies—as well as to reduce the risks involved, such as changes made as a result of Jesse Gelsinger's death (see chapter 4)—have increased dramatically. In a 2018 perspective piece, Francis Collins of the NIH and Scott Gottlieb of the FDA acknowledge both how far the field has come as well as the potential it still has:[16]

> In the view of the senior leaders of the FDA and the NIH, there is no longer sufficient evidence to claim that the risks of gene therapy are entirely unique and unpredictable—or that the field still requires special oversight that falls outside our existing framework for ensuring safety. Although scientific and safety challenges do remain—improving gene-transfer and gene-editing efficiencies, addressing immune responses and cytokine release syndrome, and in the

case of gene editing, delivery and off-target effects—the robust clinical research oversight system already accommodates for the fact that each field of research has associated unique challenges. Even as our understanding of gene therapy has advanced, so has our general framework for medical product safety. The tools we use to address other areas of science are now well suited to gene therapy.

This acknowledgment of the need to streamline the regulatory process from two of the top officials concerned with drug development and science are not the only changes that are being made. The FDA has issued various scientific guidance documents that are intended to serve as building blocks for a framework to help advance the field of gene therapy.[17] In a press release, FDA Commissioner Gottlieb stated, "Gene therapies are being studied in many areas, including genetic disorders, autoimmune diseases, heart disease, cancer and HIV/AIDS. We look forward to working with the academic and research communities to make safe and effective products a reality for more patients."[18]

The draft guidance documents include three disease-related ones—on gene therapies to treat hemophilia, retinal disorders, and rare diseases—and three on manufacturing gene therapies. They provide recommendations for the conduct of studies where a surrogate endpoint may qualify for expedited approval. They also deal with issues such as low patient enrollment, which is the case with several rare diseases. In this instance, a well-defined natural history study has the potential to be used for comparison, as it was for spinal muscular atrophy type 1 and AveXis's gene therapy product. Safety will always remain a key priority in the development of these powerful therapies, particularly when adding the ability to permanently edit the human genome into the mix. Now, not only can we read and understand the dictionary of the human genome, but we can also change its words and sentences.

With all the new therapies that are being designed, the FDA is encouraging their developers to engage in a dialogue with the agency early on in the process, in order to "refashion our traditional tools for regulation to meet the challenges and opportunities presented by such highly innovative products as cell-based regenerative medicine."[19] More than 700 proposals for gene therapy and gene editing submitted to the FDA have active investigational new drug applications, so "it seems reasonable to envision a day when gene therapy will be a mainstay of treatment for many diseases."[20]

≡ There is palpable optimism that its effectiveness in treating blood-based "liquid" tumors can translate into an ability to treat "solid" tumors, such as lung, prostate, breast, and colon cancer. With gene therapy, the hope is that its reach will extend to several other diseases in the eye, liver, muscles, central nervous system, blood, heart, and brain. The gene-editing phenomenon has exploded with the exploration of CRISPR-based technologies, and these will transform therapeutics. What follows is a snapshot of the strategies that may lead to future breakthroughs.

In addition to the progress seen in both acute lymphoblastic leukemia and diffuse large B-cell lymphoma with CD19-targeted CAR-T therapies, CAR-T therapies targeting B-cell maturation antigens (BCMA) in the treatment of multiple myeloma (a "liquid" cancer formed by malignant plasma cells found in the bone marrow) are showing robust results. Moreover, patients treated with BCMA-targeted CAR-T cells in clinical trials to date have late-stage, relapsed/refractory multiple myeloma, meaning their cancer had still progressed after receiving an average of 7 or 8 treatment regimens that were available for the disease prior to enrolling in the study.

Bristol Myers and bluebird bio developed one of the longest studied BCMA-targeted CAR-T products, called bb2121. At the

2018 annual meeting of the American Society of Clinical Oncology (ASCO) in Chicago, Illinois. Noopur Raje, director of the Multiple Myeloma Center at Massachusetts General Hospital, presented results from a Phase I study with bb2121.[21] They showed that patients receiving a dose above 150 million genetically modified cells had an overall response rate of 95.5 percent, and this treatment delayed the progression of disease by almost 1 year in the average patient. This "illustrates BCMA as a promising target in this incurable disease," noted Raje. The product, now an FDA-approved therapy called Abecma (idecabtagene vicleucel, or idecel for short),[22] showed a 73.4 percent response rate in patients receiving a dose of 150–450 million cells in a pivotal Phase II trial.[23]

Next-generation companies focused on cell immunotherapy are forming at a rapid rate. Some familiar faces from this volume are continuing the push to determine the full potential of this novel approach. Carl June is involved in the development of several next-generation T cell immunotherapies.[24] Arie Belldegrun and his colleague from Kite Pharma, David Chang, aim to create the next generation of T cell therapies with a new company, in order to "take the same biological processes that allow the first-generation autologous CAR T therapies to deliver breakthrough clinical benefits, but eliminate the need to create a personalized therapy for each patient."[25] Instead, the idea is to start with T cells from healthy donors, which will create an "off-the-shelf" inventory of cells for use in patients that will be faster, more reliable, and happen at greater scale. Bob Nelsen has funded various companies in the cell therapy, gene therapy, and gene-editing spaces, in the belief that the future of cell therapy could include vials of different cell types in every hospital that are targeted to the specific signatures not just of types of cancer, but other medical conditions, including in cardiovascular, neurodegenerative, and autoimmune diseases. He refers to it as "a cell apothecary."

Gene therapy with adeno-associated viruses continues to show promising data for diseases associated with a single gene mutation, also referred to as a monogeneic disorder. These include several liver, eye, and neurological disorders. In June 2018, early results were promising for three children with Duchenne muscular dystrophy (DMD) who were treated with an AAV gene therapy containing a gene the encodes a microdystrophin protein (a shorter version of a full-length dystrophin protein).[26] As Jerry Mendell noted, "I have been waiting my entire 49-year career to find a therapy that dramatically reduces CK [creatinine kinase] levels and creates significant levels of dystrophin. Although the data are early and preliminary, these results, if they persist and are confirmed in additional patients, will represent an unprecedented advancement in the treatment of DMD. I look forward to treating more patients in the clinical study to generate the data necessary to bring this therapy to patients with DMD, with the goal of dramatically changing the course of the disease." The *in vivo* gene therapy field continues to grow in both the size and scope of what is possible with AAV, as well as in other nonviral gene therapies being developed to potentially improve on the results seen to date.

In a blog post on sickle cell anemia, Francis Collins said, "I'm heartened to report that, thanks to decades of biomedical advances, we stand on the verge of a cure for SCD."[27] Experts are hopeful that a programmatic approach to supporting innovation and refining current technologies will lead to a breakthrough on a par with those seen in a patient treated with *ex vivo* gene therapy in Paris and Victoria Gray's treatment with the CRISPR-edited gene therapy CTX001 (see chapter 6). The NIH's National Heart, Lung, and Blood Institute's Cure Sickle Cell Initiative includes the following:[28]

- providing assistance to investigators in how to navigate the federal regulatory process,

- strengthening the input of patients and families in the design and implementation of clinical trials and novel treatments,
- directing support to technical advancements aimed at making novel approaches more universally available, and
- encouraging novel endpoints and clinical trial designs.

In addition to the initial success of *ex vivo* CRISPR-Cas9–based therapy in sickle cell disease, in June 2021, a presentation at the Peripheral Nerve Society's Annual Meeting and a concurrent publication in the *New England Journal of Medicine* reported the first clinical evidence of the safety and effectiveness of *in vivo* gene editing using CRISPR-Cas9.[29] These interim results included data from the Phase I trial of Intellia Therapeutics and Regeneron Pharmaceuticals' gene-editing therapy for the treatment of transthyretin (ATTR) amyloidosis, a rare hereditary disease characterized by the buildup of abnormal deposits of a protein (amyloidosis) in the body's organs and tissues.[30] The data were widely viewed as a resounding success, highlighting a proof-of-concept that CRISPR-Cas9 could be delivered directly into a human patient and achieve a meaningful therapeutic benefit.

The potential to create one-time, long-lasting treatments has never been more real. In the future, these may not be restricted merely to monogenic disorders, but may also work in chronic diseases, such as diabetes. As Walter Isaacson notes in *The Code Breaker*, "For the first time in the evolution of life on this planet, a species has developed to capacity to edit its own genomic makeup. That offers the potential of wondrous benefits, including the elimination of many deadly diseases and debilitating abnormalities. And it will someday offer both the promise and peril of allowing us, or some of us, to boost our bodies and enhance our babies to have better muscles, minds, memory, and moods."[31] The genomic revolution has the potential to impact human health by offering more efficient and effective health care, fewer surgeries, and longer life. Nonetheless, ethical questions abound concerning what should be its "red line"—that is, the furthest limit of what can be tolerated.

With the discoveries over the last several decades of scientific research, we are clearly entering a rapid growth phase of innovation that is catalyzed by the broadening intersection of "Health Care" and "Technology" Streets. As we continue to gain an understanding of what the true drivers of disease are—as well as how we can either prevent them from occurring or treat them—the greater the role specific, targeted therapies are likely to play in drug development. As we look ahead to potential health care challenges—for example, the growing childhood obesity epidemic and the increase in neurological disorders, such as Alzheimer's disease or Parkinson's disease—we must continue to focus on biotechnology innovations and provide an environment in which to explore what's possible. In this way, we can build a framework that will catalyze the discovery of future breakthroughs.

Epilogue
COVID-19

Sometimes there has to be a breakdown before there can be a breakthrough. On January 9, 2020, the World Health Organization announced a spate of pneumonia-like cases in Wuhan, China, which had begun in December 2019 and stemmed from a new coronavirus, which would soon be called SARS-CoV-2, or Severe Acute Respiratory Syndrome Coronavirus 2. Human coronaviruses were first identified in the mid-1960s, and some can easily infect people, accounting for 5 to 30 percent of common colds. Coronaviruses also infect animals and can evolve to make people sick, which could then lead to outbreaks of disease in humans. Previous examples in history include SARS-CoV-1 (Severe Acute Respiratory Syndrome Coronavirus 1) and MERS-CoV (Middle East Respiratory Syndrome Coronavirus).[1]

SARS-CoV-1 first emerged in Foshan, China, in November 2002, with several instances of transmission to countries such as Taiwan and Singapore. No additional infected human cases have been reported since May 2004, however.[2] MERS-CoV first occurred in April 2012 in Jordan, with all cases linked to travel to or residence in countries near the Arabian Peninsula.[3] Highlighting the devastating impact of infection, the Centers for Disease Control and Prevention reports that "about 3 or 4 out of every 10 patients reported with MERS have died."[4]

With the backdrop of potential risks related to coronaviruses that can be transmitted among people, combined with outbreaks of other viral diseases—for example, Ebola in West Africa, the Zika virus in the Asia-Pacific region and the Americas, and H1N1 influenza—some experts warned of potential unpreparedness for a global pandemic. In a May 31, 2018, article in the *New England Journal of Medicine*, Bill Gates noted, "Yet there is one area where the world isn't making much progress: pandemic preparedness. This failure should concern us all, because history has taught us there will be another deadly global pandemic. We can't predict when, but given the continual emergence of new pathogens, the increasing risk of a bioterror attack, and the ever-increasing connectedness of our world, there is a significant probability that a large and lethal modern-day pandemic will occur in our lifetime."[5]

Despite the warnings of hypothetical scenarios, the length and depth of the shock arising from COVID-19, a disease caused by SARS-CoV-2, was unexpected. The full human cost of the ongoing pandemic to the world at large is now truly incalculable. By February 2020, the COVID-19 Dashboard, from the Coronavirus Resource Center at Johns Hopkins University & Medicine, became an indispensable resource to track the worldwide infection and death rates.[6] Each day, the number of global cases would increase, with its bright red font beaming from the screen, almost ingraining itself on the reader's retina. Its world map, which started out with only few red dots, continued to fill up. No continent was off limits. The global death toll, exceeding 5.5 million as of January 2022, shows just a fraction of the whole story. Everybody has had to make sacrifices, with the immeasurable suffering of loved ones and lost memories contributing a solemn under-pinning to the overall disruption of society.

A variety of responses arose during this time:

- Local and national governments instituted public health and social distancing measures (some states and countries were more successful than others).
- The supply of personal protective equipment and testing capacity issues became a major focal point of popular press coverage.
- Phrases such as "flatten the curve" became part of the common vocabulary.
- The use of masks generated a political discussion (at least in the United States), with those refusing to wear them not acknowledging the clear scientific consensus to do so.

In addition, the drug development industry instituted a three-pronged attack for treatments of this virus: (1) antivirals and re-purposed drugs, (2) antibody therapy, and (3) vaccines.

The first potential sign of success came on April 29, 2020, when Gilead Sciences' remdesivir, an antiviral drug originally developed for SARS-CoV-1 and MERS-CoV, met the primary endpoint of the COVID-19 trial conducted by the National Institute of Allergy and Infectious Diseases: time to recovery (defined as achieving no necessity for supplemental oxygen and medical care in a hospital setting, requiring home oxygen and reduced activities, or needing neither hospitalization nor limitations on activities).[7] The drug reduced the median period that severely ill, hospitalized COVID-19 patients required to recover.

Two days after the interim results from this study (called the Adaptive Covid-19 Treatment Trial, or ACTT-1) were released, the FDA granted emergency use authorization (EUA) for remdesivir in patients with severe COVID-19 symptoms.[8] An ACTT-2 trial was instituted in May 2020. By November, it showed that Eli

Lilly's barcitinib, when added to remdesivir, was superior to rem-desivir alone in further reducing recovery time and accelerating improvement among patients with COVID-19, especially for those receiving high-flow oxygen or noninvasive ventilation.[9] On November 19, 2020, the FDA granted EUA for barcitinib, in combination with remdesivir, for the treatment of suspected or laboratory-confirmed COVID-19 in hospitalized adults and pediatric patients 2 years of age or older requiring supplemental oxygen, invasive mechanical ventilation, or "extracorporeal membrane oxygenation" (to provide cardiac and respiratory support).[10]

In June 2020, the RECOVERY (Randomised Evaluation of COVID-19 Therapy) Collaborative Group in the United Kingdom found a positive response to dexamethasone, a low-cost steroid used since the 1960s to reduce inflammation in diseases ranging from endocrine disorders to skin disease to some cancers. Their data, published in July 2020, showed that a daily administration of 6 milligrams of dexamethasone for 10 days decreased 28-day mortality rates by approximately one-third in ventilated COVID-19 patients and one-fifth in patients receiving only supplemental oxygen, but not among those receiving no respiratory support.[11]

The above therapeutic methods all used repurposed drugs, which could be tested almost immediately. To create more sophisticated treatments for the virus, however, investigators had to understand how COVID-19 infects people. On January 10, 2020, researchers published the SARS-CoV-2 virus sequence.[12] One important finding, derived from the sequencing and structural identification of the virus, was that the virus's coat contains multiple proteins, including a spike (S) protein that allows the virus to attach to, enter, and replicate within host cells. The virus is then either shed out of the infected cell and into its noninfected neighbors or released through the body's mucus membranes.

For common infections that do not result in death, the human immune system naturally produces antibodies that serve as a defense mechanism. Monoclonal antibody therapies are already used in several current treatments on the market for diseases such as cancer (e.g., Merck's Keytruda) and rheumatic disorders (e.g., AbbVie's Humira). These neutralizing antibodies are engineered to target a specific receptor and are usually delivered intravenously. In the case of COVID-19, the antibody therapy targets the S protein.

In September 2020, Eli Lilly announced that the results of an interim analysis of its Phase II Blaze-1 study of bamlanivimab (in mild to moderately ill patients who recently developed symptoms) represented a move toward treating patients earlier in the course of the disease, before they progressed to being severe ill or required hospitalization.[13] In October 2020, Regeneron announced impressive results from an additional 524 patients in the Phase II/III study of its antibody cocktail, REGN-COV2. Treatment with REGN-COV2 reduced COVID-19 related medical visits by 57 percent in the overall population, and by 72 percent in patients with at least one risk factor for a severe form of the disease.[14]

Both products received emergency use authorization, and the companies were able to produce doses on the order of hundreds of thousands.[15,16] The shortfall in supply, as well as the cost of producing these drugs, made it difficult to distribute them nationally to millions, not to mention globally to billions. That task could only be fulfilled by the third category of treatments: vaccines.

☰ Vaccines exploit the human immune system's ability to respond to and remember encounters with pathogens it recognizes as foreign to the body. Conventional methods for developing vaccines include using a live attenuated (i.e., weakened or inactivated) virus to product a strong immune response, but not enough to cause significant disease symptoms. There is a trade-off in how much of the attenuated virus can be given, so some currently approved vaccines require multiple doses. Vaccines have the ability to produce antibodies, as well as T cell responses, that contribute to the durable immune protection they offer against the targeted pathogen. Vaccines have transformed public health, with the World Health Organization noting that millions of lives are saved each year by current immunization programs.[17]

As of December 2020, there were roughly 57 vaccine candidates for COVID-19 in clinical trials, and at least 86 vaccine candidates in preclinical development. The majority sought to offer protection against either the S protein or specific parts of it that are recognized by the immune system, using multiple vaccine models. The theory was that if a vaccine can generate a robust neutralizing antibody and a memory response to the S protein in a host cell, then that host cell will be able to combat the S protein mechanism of SARS-CoV-2 and confer immunity against COVID-19, as well as prevent the spread of the virus itself.

Operation Warp Speed was a public-private partnership initiated by the US government to accelerate the development, manufacture, and distribution of COVID-19 vaccines, therapeutics, and diagnostics. As its head, Moncef Slaoui explained, "The way we decided [which vaccines to include in Operation Warp Speed] was to say first, we should have a portfolio of products, not just one or two. Second, we should diversify the biological risk by using different platform technologies, different approaches to designing a vaccine, because we are not sure which one is going to work. Third, we're going to diversify the execution risk and the much more granular details within each one of the technologies selected by making sure we have two representatives in each technology."[18]

The vaccines that led the global development landscape utilized messenger RNA (mRNA) technology, which instructs cells in the body to make the virus's spike protein. This triggers the immune system to develop a defense mechanism that can recognize the infection. In the body, mRNAs function as temporary instruction manuals, created to help cells make proteins and then degraded shortly thereafter. This process can be thought of as the "software of life," integral to the central precept of biology. DNA serves as a hard drive, storing instructions for specific proteins. The proteins are the software applications, allowing particular functions in the human body, encoded by DNA and communicated by mRNA. DNA has four major building blocks—adenine, thymine, guanine, and cytosine—as well as a double helix structure, whereas mRNA is uses uracil instead of thymine, while maintaining the other three, usually in a single strand.

In May 1961, two articles were published in the journal *Nature* that discussed the isolation of mRNA and provided an argument for its role in gene regulation.[19,20] The two research groups used slightly different techniques to assess the problem from different angles—part of the basic scientific research process that builds the foundational understanding on which breakthroughs are formed—but both arrived at a similar conclusion.

One of the drivers of the use of mRNA as a therapeutic method was Katalin Karikó, at the University of Pennsylvania School of Medicine. She first became interested in mRNA as an alternative to DNA-based therapy to alleviate some of the long-time safety concerns with gene therapy. In 2005, Karikó, Drew Weissman, and two other colleagues published a study where they replaced one of mRNA's building blocks, uracil, thus allowing the modified mRNA to evade the body's immune system. She presciently predicted, "Insights gained from this study could advance our understanding of autoimmune diseases where nucleic acids play a prominent role in the pathogenesis, determine a role for nucleoside modifications in viral RNA, and give future directions into the design of therapeutic RNAs."[21]

Ugun Sahin was another instrumental player. He was born in Iskenderum, Turkey, and moved to Cologne, Germany, when he was four years old. Sahin later became a physician at the University of Cologne. Early in his career, he met and married Ozlem Tureci, the daughter of a Turkish physician. She had immigrated to Germany from Istanbul. In 2001, the two started Ganymed Pharmaceuticals, a company developing monoclonal antibodies to treat cancer. Astellas Pharma acquired Ganymed for €422 million in 2016.[22] In 2008, the couple founded BioNTech, initially focused "on the understanding that every cancer patient's tumor is unique and therefore each patient's treatment should be individualized."[23]

On March 13, 2020, Pfizer signaled its five-point plan to battle COVID-19:[24]

1. sharing tools and insights,
2. marshaling our people,
3. applying our drug development expertise,
4. offering our manufacturing capabilities, and
5. improving future rapid response.

Four days later, Pfizer and BioNTech announced their intent to jointly develop the latter's mRNA-based vaccine candidate, BNT162, to prevent COVID-19 infections.[25] This collaboration built on a previous 2018 agreement the two firms had signed to codevelop an mRNA-based influenza vaccine. Progress in developing this new vaccine moved forward rapidly.[26] On April 22, 2020, the companies announced approval from the Paul-Ehrlich-Institut, the German regulatory authority, to commence a Phase I/II clinical trial for their COVID-19 vaccine program.[27]

In the United States, a team led by Derrick Rossi, then at Boston Children's Hospital in Massachusetts, published a study in 2010 where modified mRNA was used to encode proteins that reprogrammed adult cells into embryonic-like stem cells, building on the work of Shinya Yamanaka.[28] (In 2012, Yamanaka was a corecipient of the Nobel Prize in Physiology or Medicine.)[29] Rossi's fellow colleagues, Kenneth Chien and Robert Langer (a well-known, prolific entrepreneur in his own right), joined Derrick in pitching this scientific advance, using it as the basis for a stem cell company, to the venture creation firm Flagship Pioneering. Flagship's CEO, Noubar Afeyan, founded the company in 2000 as "an enterprise where entrepreneurially minded scientists invent seemingly unreasonable solutions to challenges facing human health and sustainability," beginning by asking the question "What if?" and then finding an answer ("It turns out that").[30]

Langer, Rossi, Chen, and Afeyan founded a company that was based on the premise of exploring mRNA as a potential new class of medicines. Initially called "Flagship NewCo LS18," it later become Moderna.[31] Here, according to Afeyan, the three "what ifs" were:

1. What if patients could make their own biotherapeutics?
2. What if this process could be transient, controllable, multipotent, and safe?
3. What if the cost and time for new candidate selection and testing could be dramatically reduced?

Prior to the onset of the COVID-19 pandemic, Moderna, with CEO Stéphane Bancel at the helm, had defined itself as pioneering mRNA therapeutics and vaccines to create a new generation of transformative medicines. On January 13, 2020, following the publication two days earlier of the SARS-CoV-2 sequence and structure,[12] scientists at Moderna and the Vaccine Research Center (VRC), part of NIH's National Institute of Allergy and Infectious Diseases, finalized the sequence for a vaccine candidate called mRNA-1273.[32]

As Stéphane Bancel recalls, "the VRC and Moderna teams separately designed the sequence for the vaccine candidate within 48 hours and both had independently come up with the same design for mRNA-1273." The speed with which they were able to develop this was partially due prior collaboration between the two on a MERS-CoV vaccine candidate.[33] As Barney Graham, a key scientist on the VRC team, notes, "New manufacturing platforms, structure-based antigen design, computational biology, protein engineering, and gene synthesis have provided the tools to now make vaccines with speed and precision."[34]

On May 18, 2020, Moderna announced positive interim Phase I results with mRNA-1273, the first vaccine data that showed the potential to produce neutralizing antibodies against the virus.[35] Tal Zaks, Moderna's chief medical officer noted that, "When combined with the success in preventing viral replication in the lungs of a pre-clinical challenge model at a dose that elicited similar levels of neutralizing antibodies, these data substantiate our belief that mRNA-1273 has the potential to prevent COVID-19 disease and advance our ability to select a dose for pivotal trial." On July 1, 2020, Pfizer and BioNTech announced early positive data from a Phase I/II study of BNT162b1, the most advanced of four investigational candidates from their BNT162 program.[36] On July 27, both Pfizer/BioNTech and Moderna initiated their late-stage, placebo-controlled Phase II/III clinical trials, which would have the potential to lead to regulatory approval for their vaccines. Pfizer and BioNTech advanced their BNT162b2 vaccine candidate into a Phase II/III study at a 30-microgram dose level in a two-dose regimen.[37] The Moderna Phase III (COVE) trial, conducted in collaboration with the Biomedical Advanced Research and Development Authority (part of the US Department of Health and Human Services) and the NIH, was also a randomized, placebo-controlled trial testing a two-dose regiment of 100 micrograms of mRNA-1273.[38]

These late-stage trials were not without their ups and downs, particularly in relation to scientific integrity and the need to enroll representative populations, reflecting real-world use of the vaccines, in the trials. With regard to assuring the public of their focus on maintaining rigorous scientific integrity in their studies, the CEOs of Moderna, BioNTech, and Pfizer, along with the CEOs of six other biotechnology companies developing COVID-19 vaccines, signed a pledge to "make clear our on-going commitment to developing and testing potential vaccines for COVID-19 in accordance with high ethical standards and sound scientific principles," as well as comply with the following verbatim statements:[39]

- Always make the safety and well-being of vaccinated individuals our top priority.
- Continue to adhere to high scientific and ethical standards regarding the conduct of clinical trials and the rigor of manufacturing processes.
- Only submit [vaccine candidates] for approval or emergency use authorization after demonstrating safety and efficacy through a Phase 3 clinical study that is designed and conducted to meet requirements of expert regulatory authorities such as [the] FDA.
- Work to ensure a sufficient supply and range of vaccine options, including those suitable for global access.

In September 2020, Pfizer and BioNTech expanded the enrollment in their trial to up to 44,000 participants, to "include adolescents as young as 16 years of age and people with chronic, stable HIV, Hepatitis C, or Hepatitis B infection, as well as provide additional safety and efficacy data."[40] Moderna also slowed down its trial enrollment that month, to ensure minority representation, since, at the time, two-thirds of those in the study were white, 20 percent were Hispanic or Latino, and 7 percent were black.[41] "It was the hardest decision I made this year," Bancel noted in a *New York Times* article, because it meant that Moderna would face a delay of up to three weeks and Pfizer/BioNTech would take the lead.[42] On November 9, 2020, Pfizer and BioNTech announced that BNT162b2 was more than 90 percent effective against COVID-19, based on their first interim analysis.[43] A Moderna news release on November 16 announced that mRNA-1273 had an efficacy of 94.5 percent in its COVE trial.[44]

≡ On December 10th, the FDA convened a meeting of its Vaccines and Related Biological Products Advisory Committee (VRBPAC)—an event similar to those described in the chapters on previous breakthroughs, albeit conducted virtually this time—to discuss an emergency use authorization for the Pfizer-BioNTech COVID-19 vaccine.[45] The question under consideration was, "Based on the totality of scientific evidence available, do the benefits of the Pfizer-BioNTech COVID-19 vaccine outweigh its risks for use in individuals 16 years of age and older?" The VRBPAC voted 17 to 4 in favor, with one member abstaining.[46]

In their commentary, committee members were overwhelmingly positive about the effectiveness of the vaccine, although some were concerned about the inclusion of 16- and 17-year-olds in the EUA, given that there was less safety data on this population. There were also reports of allergic reactions in two individuals in the United Kingdom who received the vaccine. The committee members also sought more information about the potential of the vaccine to reduce transmission of the disease and sought clarity on the timing of additional data, which Pfizer expected to have in early 2021. Pfizer also noted that it needed six months of follow-up data for a full biological license application to the FDA.

On December 17, the VRBPAC met again to discuss an emergency use authorization for Moderna's vaccine.[47] The committee voted 20 to 0 in favor, with one abstention, to the question, "Based on the totality of scientific evidence available, do the benefits of the Moderna COVID-19 Vaccine outweigh its risks for use in individuals 18 years of age and older?" Committee members were overwhelmingly positive on the benefit-risk profile of the vaccine. The only issue raised was over concerns related to Moderna's plans to "unblind" its ongoing Phase III study [where all participants would receive the treatment, rather than having some only get a placebo] and vaccinate trial participants after the FDA issued an EUA, which would limit the study's ability to capture long-term efficacy and safety data.

Granting an Emergency Use Authorization to Moderna added approximately 20 million vaccine doses for the United States by the end of 2020, roughly doubling the available amount of vaccine available. Moreover, compared with Pfizer's vaccine, Moderna's has less stringent handling requirements, can be stored in standard medical freezers, and has smaller minimum order requirements, which would enable broader distribution of the vaccine to rural areas, which are less well-equipped to handle Pfizer's ultracold storage temperatures (−94° F) and larger minimum order requirements.[48,49]

In 2020, the United States granted emergency use authorization of the two vaccines developed by Pfizer-BioNTech (December 11) and Moderna (December 18) following their respective advisory committee meetings, providing an exclamation point for the fastest vaccine research and development programs in history. Pfizer's CEO, Albert Bourla, stated, "Pfizer's purpose is breakthroughs that change patients' lives, and in our 171-year history there has never been a more urgent need for a breakthrough than today with hundreds of thousands of people continuing to suffer from COVID-19. . . . As a U.S. company, today's news brings great pride and tremendous joy that Pfizer has risen to the challenge to develop a vaccine that has the potential to help bring an end to this devastating pandemic. We have worked tirelessly to make the impossible possible, steadfast in our belief that science will win."[50]

Stéphane Bancel, Moderna's CEO, noted, "We were able to create and manufacture the Moderna COVID-19 Vaccine in 11 months from sequence to authorization, while advancing clinical development with a Phase 1, Phase 2 and pivotal Phase 3 study of

30,000 participants. It has been a 10-year scientific, entrepreneurial and medical journey and I am thankful to all those who have helped us get here today. We remain focused on scaling up manufacturing to help us protect as many people as we can from this terrible disease."[51]

Noubar Afeyan, reflecting on the development of Moderna's mRNA-1273, noted that "the most gravity-defying activity was the scale up of a compound from 2000 dose capacity to 200 million dose capacity in record speed." Expansion of the foundational science behind mRNA technology for therapeutic use, the speed with which the COVID-19 vaccines were developed, and the regulatory hurdles they passed—all while under the world's microscope —highlight the potential upside of focusing global resources on building breakthroughs.

≡ The COVID-19 pandemic sparked a revolution where the timelines of my previous examples of breakthroughs were significantly shortened as scientists, the pharmaceutical industry, and governmental agencies worked at breakneck speed to understand the disease and develop safe and effective therapeutics and vaccines. While the year 2020 saw unimaginable sorrow and loss across the world, it also saw rapid advances in understanding the biology, origination, development, and clinical characteristics of this infectious disease. Certain areas of red tape were cut to propel the full innovative engine that underlies the biotechnology industry. The overarching themes of building breakthroughs discussed in this book were prevalent in the development of the mRNA vaccines by Pfizer/BioNTech and Moderna.

The underlying science of messenger RNA as a therapeutic treatment started around the time of Karikó, Weismann and colleagues' 2005 discovery that modified mRNA could evade the body's immune system.[21] What followed were lessons in persisting, learning from failure, and building an environment that promoted "outside the box" thinking, discussed and exemplified in this book by chapters on the development of CAR-T therapy, *in vivo* gene therapy, and *ex vivo* gene-corrected cell therapy. In addition to the scientific foundation for these developments, venture capital and entrepreneurship were important in translating this science into new firms that could revolutionize the vaccine-manufacturing process. Lastly, these mRNA companies had the wherewithal to change course, switching to a focus on developing what would become the first two approved COVID-19 vaccines in the United States.

COVID-19 is not the first pandemic that humanity has faced, and it will not be the last. With new variants that have arisen, such as Delta and Omicron, COVID-19 is more aptly called an endemic—that is, an infection that is constantly maintained at a baseline level in a geographic area, which, in this case, is throughout the globe. Two of the key ingredients in Operation Warp Speed's success were educated intuition—an anchored set of knowledge and experience that drives the approach to a problem in the right direction—and the intrinsic alignment of all constituencies, which happens particularly well in crises. As Moncef Slaoui noted, "each company maintained their intellectual property. Yet everything else was shared—in how you conduct a clinical trial, how you build a manufacturing site, how you recruit [different types of patients] . . . how to measure the immune response. Everything that wasn't in the product itself, the collaboration and openness was maximal. . . . So it is possible actually to maintain the area that's competitive and then identify everything else that's not."[18] The building blocks of collaboration and competition were key.

≡ Continuing to innovate is imperative in building breakthroughs, in order to have a deeper fundamental understanding of health and disease, create novel discovery tools, find new means to control biology, and analyze large datasets. In the case of Moderna's COVID-19 vaccine, it took an enormous bet of roughly $2.5 billion in private and public capital (the building blocks of perseverance, incentivization, and social capital), conviction about the initial concept (the building block of the big idea), the creation of a digital platform for the work (the building block of never stop learning), and a culture of dedication to the project (the building block of building an environment that promotes thinking 'outside the box').

From a health care perspective, what we have learned from this endemic should further accelerate developments and investments in medicine as a whole, not just against future pandemics. As Noubar Afeyan summarizes, "We now know that certain things can be done, society does not need to accept, and should not accept, 40,000 to 50,000 influenza deaths per year or a six-year vaccine development. We can find ways to take the learnings from the pandemic and apply them selectively and judiciously to a lot of other areas. The more good that this experience can allow us to bring to other aspects of health, the better the meaning of the all these sacrifices would be."

Acknowledgments

Finishing a project like this allows you to take stock of all the people that helped you along the way, and there are so many people that I'd like to thank. First, I'm grateful to my editor Robin Coleman, the peer reviewers that gave their time to critique earlier drafts of this manuscript, and the copyediting (special thanks to freelancer Kathleen Capels) and marketing teams at Johns Hopkins University Press. At the outset, I don't think I would've expected nearly six years of emails, edits, rewrites, and hundreds of drafts, but the finished product was better because of it. I appreciate all the hard work.

Thank you to everyone who took the time to speak with me and provide many of the quotations in this book. First, the patients and their families: Tom, Kari, and Emily Whitehead; Emily Dumler; Nicole, Derwin, and Matteo Almeida; and Terry Jackson. Second, individuals at the Emily Whitehead Foundation, SMA Foundation, and the Foundation for Sickle Cell Disease Research and Sickle Cell Care and Research Network. Additionally, I would like to salute the physicians who took the time to discuss these examples of breakthroughs, particularly Carl June, Jerry Mendell, Thomas Crawford, Katherine High, Michael Jensen, and Maria Cavazzana. Thanks to the entrepreneurs and venture capitalists who took the time to give me a look into the investing and company formation process: Robert Nelsen at ARCH Venture Partners; Bruce Booth at Atlas Ventures; Bob More at Alta Partners; Noubar Afeyan, Christine Heenan, and Andrew LaPrade at Flagship Pioneering; and Arie Belldegrun, David Chang, and Christine Cassiano at Allogene Therapeutics / Vida Ventures. I would also be remiss if I didn't recognize several sources that provided consistent background research citations for this book: *Science*, *Nature*, the *New England Journal of Medicine*, *Forbes*, the *New York Times*, the *Wall Street Journal*, the STAT News website, and the LifeSci VC blog, among others.

A sincere thank you to all my current and former William Blair & Company colleagues and the whole biotechnology equity research team. The mentorship and collegiality at the firm and within our team has been critical to my development, both professionally and personally. A special nod of appreciation to John Flavin, Portal Innovations, and Fulton Labs for involving me in the plan to grow a biotech innovation hub in the Midwest. My gratitude, as well, to my academic mentors: David DeMarini, Rebecca Fry, Carl Blackman, David Edwards, and Jorge Muñiz Ortiz.

My greatest appreciation goes to my family. My wife, Lindsey, continues to be the most supportive partner and an inspiration for everything I do. My daughters, Maya and Neela, have already provided me with more joy in my life than I could have ever imagined and continue to amaze me every single day. My mother, Geetha, and late father, M. G. Prasad, always instilled in us the importance of education and a love for the arts. My brother, Teju, has led by example in continuing to pursue his passions. I am grateful to my brother-in-law and sister-in-law, Michael and Julie

Vaccaro, for their support in reading the manuscript and providing commentary as well as to my extended family. Big salutes to three of my literary "muses," Barack Obama, Jay-Z, and Lin-Manuel Miranda, for giving me the motivation I needed to move forward in all my pursuits. Lastly, thanks to my childhood friends—Amit, Emilio, Anthony, Van, and Paul—who always keep me grounded.

References

Introduction

1. Isaacson W. Should the rich be allowed to buy the best genes? AirMail News. July 27, 2019. https://airmail.news/issues/2019-7-27/should-the-rich-be-allowed-to-buy-the-best-genes/.
2. Obama B. President Obama's 2016 State of the Union address. Obama White House. January 12, 2016. https://medium.com/@ObamaWhiteHouse/president-obama-s-2016-state-of-the-union-address-7c06300f9726/.
3. Kennedy JF. Excerpt from special message to the Congress on urgent national needs. Speech delivered in person before a joint session of Congress. NASA History. May 25, 1961. https://www.nasa.gov/vision/space/features/jfk_speech_text.html.
4. For definitions of various FDA terms and abbreviations used in this book, see US Food and Drug Administration. Drugs@FDA glossary of terms. https://www.fda.gov/drugs/drug-approvals-and-databases/drugsfda-glossary-terms/.
5. Thomas DW, Burna J, Audette J, Carroll A, Dow-Hygelund C, Hay M. *Clinical Development Success Rates 2006–2015.* Biotechnology Innovation Organization. 2016. https://www.bio.org/sites/default/files/leg

acy/bioorg/docs/Clinical%20Development%20Success%20Rates%20
2006-2015%20-%20BIO,%20Biomedtracker,%20Amplion%202016
.pdf.

6. Glenner GG, Wong CW. Alzheimer's disease: initial report of the puri-
fication and characterization of a novel cerebrovascular amyloid protein. *Biochemical and Biophysical Research Communications*. 1984;120(3):
885-890.

7. Games D, Adams D, Alessandrini R, et al. Alzheimer-type neuropath-
ology in transgenic mice overexpressing V717F beta-amyloid precursor
protein. *Nature*. 1995;373(6514):523–527.

8. Kolata G. An Alzheimer's treatment fails: "we don't have anything now."
New York Times. February 10. 2020. https://www.nytimes.com/2020/02
/10/health/alzheimers-amyloid-drug.html.

9. Begley S. The maddening saga of how an Alzheimer's "cabal" thwarted
progress toward a cure for decades. STAT News. June 25, 2019. https://
www.statnews.com/2019/06/25/alzheimers-cabal-thwarted-progress
-toward-cure/.

10. McGinley L. Furor rages over FDA approval of controversial Alzheimer's
drug, *Washington Post*. June 17, 2021. https://www.washingtonpost.com
/health/2021/06/17/alzheimers-drug-controversy/.

11. Smietana K, Siatkowski N, Moller M. Trends in clinical success rates.
Nature Reviews Drug Discovery. 2016;15(6):379–380.

chapter 1 **Leukemia and Lymphoma**

1. American Cancer Society. Cancer facts & figures 2022. https://www
.cancer.org/content/dam/cancer-org/research/cancer-facts-and-statis
tics/annual-cancer-facts-and-figures/2022/2022-cancer-facts-and
-figures.pdf.

2. Mukherjee S. *The Emperor of All Maladies: A Biography of Cancer*.
Simon & Schuster; 1983: 6–7.

3. Childhood cancer. In: Howlader N, Noone AM, Krapcho M, et al., eds.
SEER Cancer Statistics Review, 1975–2010. National Cancer Institute;
2013: Section 28. https://seer.cancer.gov/archive/csr/1975_2010/.

4. Childhood cancer by the ICCC [Inernational Calssification of Child-
hood Cancer]. In: Howlader N, Noone AM, Krapcho M, et al., eds. *SEER
Cancer Statistics Review, 1975–2010*. National Cancer Institute; 2013:
Section 29. https://seer.cancer.gov/archive/csr/1975_2010/.

5. *Fortune* magazine. *Cancer: The Great Darkness*. Doubleday, Doran; 1937.

6. Wills L. The nature of the haemopoietic factor in marmite. *Lancet*. 1933; 221(5729):1283–1286.

7. Farber S, Diamond LK, Mercer RD, et al. Temporary remissions in acute leukemia in children produced by folic acid antagonist, 4-aminopteroyl-glutamic acid 374. *New England Journal of Medicine*. 1948;238(23): 787–793.

8. Pui CH, Evans WE. A 50-year journey to cure childhood acute lymphoblastic leukemia. *Seminars in Hematology*. 2013;50(3):185–196.

9. Frei E, Freireich EJ, Gehan E, et al. Studies of sequential and combination antimetabolite therapy in acute leukemia: 6-mercaptopurine and methotrexate. *Blood*. 1961;18:431–454.

10. Pinkel D. Five-year follow-up of "total therapy" of childhood lymphocytic leukemia. *JAMA: Journal of the American Medical Association*. 1971;216:648–652.

11. Aur RJ, Simone J, Hustu HO, et al. Central nervous system therapy and combination chemotherapy of childhood lymphocytic leukemia. *Blood*. 1971;37(3):272–281.

12. American Cancer Society. Treatment of children with acute lymphocytic leukemia (ALL). Last revised February 12, 2019. https://www.cancer.org/cancer/leukemia-in-children/treating/children-with-all.html.

13. Möricke A, Zimmermann M, Valsecchi MG, et al. Dexamethasone vs prednisone in induction treatment of pediatric ALL: results of the randomized trial AIEOP-BFM ALL 2000. *Blood*. 2016;127(17):2101–2012.

14. Vora A, Goulden N, Wade R, et al. Treatment reduction for children and young adults with low-risk acute lymphoblastic leukaemia defined by minimal residual disease (UKALL 2003): a randomised controlled trial. *Lancet Oncology*. 2013;14 (3):199–209.

15. Place AE, Stevenson KE, Vrooman LM, et al. Intravenous pegylated asparaginase versus intramuscular native *Escherichia coli* L-asparaginase in newly diagnosed childhood acute lymphoblastic leukaemia (DFCI 05-001): a randomised, open-label phase 3 trial. *Lancet Oncology*. 2015;16(16):1677–1690.

16. Pieters R, de Groot-Kruseman H, van der Velden V, et al. Successful therapy reduction and intensification for childhood acute lymphoblastic leukemia based on minimal residual disease monitoring: study ALL10 from the Dutch Childhood Oncology Group. *Journal of Clinical Oncology*. 2016;34(22):2591–2601.

17. National Cancer Institute. Childhood acute lymphoblastic leukemia

treatment (PDQ®)—health professional version. Updated October 7, 2021. https://www.cancer.gov/types/leukemia/hp/child-all-treatment-pdq#cit/section_1.63/.

18. Rosenbaum L. Tragedy, perseverance, and chance—the story of CAR-T therapy. *New England Journal of Medicine*. 2017;377(14):1313–1315. doi: 10.1056/NEJMp1711886.

19. Children's Hospital of Philadelphia. Relapsed leukemia: Emily's story. December 2012; updated July 2017. https://www.chop.edu/stories/relapsed-leukemia-emilys-story/.

20. Hodgkin T. On some morbid appearances of the absorbent glands and spleen. *Medico-Chirurgical Transactions*. 1832;17:68–114.

21. Rappaport H. Tumors of the haematopoeitic system. In: *Atlas of Tumor Pathology, Section 3, Fascicle 8*. United States Armed Forces Institute of Pathology; 1966: 442.

22. Conant J. How a WWII disaster—and cover-up—led to a cancer treatment breakthrough. History Stories. August 12, 2020. https://www.history.com/news/wwii-disaster-bari-mustard-gas/.

23. Goodman LS, Wintrobe MM, Dameshek W, Goodman MJ, Gilman A, McLennan MT. Nitrogen mustard therapy: use of methyl-bis (-chloroethyl) amine hydrochloride and tris (-chloroethyl) amine hydrochloride for Hodgkin's disease, lymphosarcoma, leukemia, and certain allied and miscellaneous disorders. *JAMA: Journal of the American Medical Association*. 1946;132:126–132.

24. Gilman A, Philips FS. The biological actions and therapeutic applications of the -chloroethylamines and sulfides. *Science*. 1946;103(2675):409–415.

25. DeVita VT, Chu E. A history of cancer chemotherapy. *Cancer Research*. 2008;68(21):8643–8653.

26. DeVita VT, DeVita-Raeburn E. *The Death of Cancer: After Fifty Years on the Front Lines of Medicine, a Pioneering Oncologist Reveals Why the War on Cancer Is Winnable—and How We Can Get There*. Sarah Crichton Books; 2015.

27. Coiffier B. Non-Hodgkin's lymphomas. In: Cavalli F, Hansen HH, Kaye SB, eds. *Textbook of Medical Oncology*. Martin Dunitz; 1997: 265–287.

28. DeVita VT, Canellos GP, Chabner B, Schein P, Young RC, Hubbard SM. Advanced diffuse histiocytic lymphoma, a potentially curable disease: results with combination chemotherapy. *Lancet*. 1975;305(7901):248–254.

29. Fisher RI, Gaynor ER, Dahlberg S, et al. Comparison of a standard regi-

men (CHOP) with three intensive chemotherapy regimens for advanced non-Hodgkin's lymphoma. *New England Journal of Medicine.* 1993;328(14):1002–1006.

30. Coiffier B, Lepage E, Briere J, et al. CHOP chemotherapy plus rituximab compared with CHOP alone in elderly patients with diffuse large-B-cell lymphoma. *New England Journal of Medicine.* 2002;346(4):235–242.

chapter 2 Chimeric Antigen Receptor (CAR)-T Cell Therapy

1. Jobs S. How to live before you die. TED Talk delivered at Stanford University commencement. June 2005.

2. U.S. Environmental Protection Agency. *IRIS Toxicological Review of Carbon Tetrachloride (External Review Draft).* September 1989; archived file, may be outdated. EPA/635/R-08/005A. https://cfpub.epa.gov/ncea /risk/recordisplay.cfm?deid=119546/.

3. Carroll RG, Riley JL, Levine BL, et al. Differential regulation of HIV-1 fusion cofactor expression by CD28 costimulation of CD4+ T cells. *Science.* 1997;276(5310):273–276.

4. Levine BL, Mosca JD, Riley JL, et al. Antiviral effect and *ex vivo* CD4+ T cell proliferation in HIV-positive patients as a result of CD28 costimulation. *Science.* 1996;272(5270):1939–1943.

5. Agnew V. CAR-T pioneer and noted mentor Art Weiss, MD, PhD. Helen Diller Family Comprehensive Cancer Center, University of California, San Francisco. October 15, 2019. https://cancer.ucsf.edu/news/2019 /10/15/car-t-pioneer-and-noted-mentor-art-weiss-md-phd.9796/.

6. June C. Signal transduction in T cells. *Current Opinion in Immunology.* 1991;3(3):287–293.

7. Canavan N. *A Cure Within: Scientists Unleashing the Immune System to Kill Cancer.* Cold Spring Harbor Laboratory Press; 2018.

8. Porter DL, Levine BL, Kalos M, Bagg A, June CH. Chimeric antigen receptor-modified T cells in chronic lymphoid leukemia. *New England Journal of Medicine.* 2011;365(8):725–733.

9. Kalos M, Levine BL, Porter DL, et al. T cells with chimeric receptors have potent antitumor effects and can establish memory in patients with advanced leukemia. *Science Translational Medicine.* 2011;3(95): 95ra73.

10. Grupp SA, Kalos M, Barrett D, et al. Chimeric antigen receptor-modified T cells for acute lymphoid leukemia. *New England Journal of Medicine.* 2013;368(16):1509–1518.

11. Thiel P, Masters B. *Zero to One: Notes on Startups, or How to Build the Future*. Crown Business. 2014.

12. Richtel M, Pollack A. Harnessing the U.S. taxpayer to fight cancer and make profits. *New York Times*. December 19, 2016. https://www.ny times.com/2016/12/19/health/harnessing-the-us-taxpayer-to-fight -cancer-and-make-profits.html.

13. Neelapu SS, Tummala S, Kebriaei P, et al. Chimeric antigen receptor T-cell therapy: assessment and management of toxicities. *Nature Reviews Clinical Oncology*. 2018;15(1):47–52.

14. Konrad A, ed.; reported by Szkutak R, Wolpow N. The Midas List: the world's best venture capital investors in 2021. *Forbes*. April 13, 2021. https://www.forbes.com/midas/.

15. Harper M. Inside the brain of biotech's top venture capitalist. *Forbes*. May 11, 2016. https://www.forbes.com/sites/matthewherper/2016 /05/11/rx-for-success/.

16. Epstein D. *Range*. Penguin USA; 2020.

chapter 3 **Spinal Muscular Atrophy**

1. Mayo Clinic staff. Amniocentisis. https://www.mayoclinic.org/tests -procedures/amniocentesis/about/pac-20392914/.

2. Cure SMA. About spinal muscular atrophy. https://www.curesma.org /sma/about-sma/.

3. Werdnig G. Zwei frühhinfantile hereditäre Fälle von progressiver Muskelatrophie unter dem Bilde der Dystrophie, aber auf neurotischer Grundlage. *Archiv für Psychiatrie und Nervenkrankheiten*. 1891;22(2): 437–480.

4. Hoffman J. Ueber chronische spinale Muskelatrophie im Kindesalter, auf familiärer Basis. *Deutsche Zeitschrift für Nerveneilkunde*. 1893;3: 427.

5. Huenekens EJ, Bell ET. Infantile spinal progressive muscular atrophy (Werdnig-Hoffmann): report of a case with necropsy findings. *American Journal of Diseases of Children*. 1920;20(6):496–506. doi: 10.1001 /archpedi.1920.01910300036003.

6. Lefebvre S, Burglen L, Reboullet S, et al. Identification and characterization of a spinal muscular atrophy–determining gene. *Cell*. 1995;80(1): 155–165.

7. Lorson CL, Hahnen E, Androphy EJ. A single nucleotide in the *SMN* gene regulates splicing and is responsible for spinal muscular atrophy.

Proceedings of the National Academy of Sciences of the United States of America. 1999;96(11):6307–6311.

8. Munsat T, Davies K. Spinal muscular atrophy. Workshop report from 32nd ENMC International Workshop, Naarden, The Netherlands, 10–12 March 1995. *Neuromuscular Disorders.* 1996;6(2):125–127.

9. Posada de la Paz M, Groft SC. 2010. *Rare Diseases Epidemiology.* Advances in Experimental Medicine and Biology Series vol. 686. Springer; 2010.

10. European Medicines Agency. Unmet medical need: definitions and need for clarity. EMA-Payer community meeting. September 19, 2017. https://www.ema.europa.eu/docs/en_GB/document_library/Presentation/2017/10/WC500236332.pdf.

11. Finkel RS, McDermott MP, Kaufmann P, et al. Observational study of spinal muscular atrophy type I and implications for clinical trials. *Neurology.* 2014;83(9):810–817.

12. Le TT, Pham LT, Butchbach MER, et al. *SMNΔ7*, the major product of the centromeric survival motor neuron (*SMN2*) gene, extends survival in mice with spinal muscular atrophy and associates with full-length *SMN. Human Molecular Genetics.* 2005;14(6):845–857.

13. Watson JD, Crick FH. Molecular structure of nucleic acids: a structure for deoxyribose nucleic acid. *Nature.* 1953;171(4356):737–741.

14. Avery OT, Macleod CM, McCarty M. Studies on the chemical nature of the substance inducing transformation of pneumococcal types: induction of transformation by a desoxyribonucleic acid fraction isolated from pneumococcus type III. *Journal of Experimental Medicine.* 1944;79:137–158.

15. Lundin KE, Gissberg O, Smith CIE. Oligonucleotide therapies: the past and the present. *Human Gene Therapy.* 2015;26(8):475–485.

16. Your Genome. What is the "central dogma"? https://www.yourgenome.org/facts/what-is-the-central-dogma/.

17. Morcos PA. Achieving targeted and quantifiable alteration of mRNA splicing with Morpholino oligos. *Biochemical and Biophysical Research Communications.* 2007;358(2):521–527.

18. Singh RN, Singh NN, Singh NK, Androphy EJ, inventors; University of Massachusetts, assignee. Spinal muscular atrophy (SMA) treatment via targeting of *SMN2* splice site inhibitory sequences. US Patent 7838657. November 23, 2010. (Also published as US Patent 8110560, US Patent 8586559, US Patent 9476042, US Patent 20070292408, US Patent 20100087511, US Patent 20120165394, US Patent 20140066492.)

19. Hua Y, Vickers TA, Baker BF, Bennett CF, Krainer AR. Enhancement of *SMN2* exon 7 inclusion by antisense oligonucleotides targeting the exon. *PLoS Biology.* 2007;5(4):e73.

20. Singh NN, Howell MD, Androphy EJ, Singh RN. How the discovery of ISS-N1 led to the first medical therapy for spinal muscular atrophy. *Gene Therapy.* 2017;27(9):520–526.

21. Breakthrough Initiatives. Winners of the 2019 Breakthrough Prize in life sciences, fundamental physics, and mathematics announced. https://breakthroughprize.org/News/47/.

22. Rare Disease Day. 28 February is rare disease day. https://www.rare diseaseday.org.

23. Cure SMA. Media. https://www.curesma.org/about/media/.

24. Biogen, Inc. Highlights of prescribing information: Spinraza™. 2016. https://www.accessdata.fda.gov/drugsatfda_docs/label/2016/209531lbl .pdf.

chapter 4 *In Vivo* Gene Therapy

1. Berry FB. The story of "the Berry Plan." *Bulletin of the New York Academy of Medicine.* 1976;52(3):278–282.

2. Office of Personnel, US Public Health Service. *The Commissioned Officer in the U.S. Public Health Service.* 1967. Public Health Service Publication No. 1681.

3. Klein M. The legacy of the "Yellow Berets": the Vietnam War, the doctor draft, and the NIH Associate Training Program. Unpublished manuscript. 1998. Office of NIH History and Stetten Museum. https://history .nih.gov/display/history/Publications?preview=/1016824/8883689 /YellowBerets.pdf.

4. Khot S, Park BS, Longstreth WT Jr. The Vietnam War and medical research: untold legacy of the U.S. doctor draft and the NIH "Yellow Berets." *Academic Medicine.* 2011;86(4):502–508. https://journals.lww.com/ academicmedicine/Fulltext/2011/04000/The_Vietnam_War_and _Medical_Research__Untold.25.aspx.

5. Data from NIH Associate Training Program database. Copy available on CD ROM from Office of NIH History and Stetten Museum, Bethesda, Maryland. Also see Moss GD. *Vietnam: An American Ordeal.* Prentice-Hall; 1994.

6. Ginsberg HS. The life and times of adenoviruses. *Advances in Virus Research.* 1999;54:1–13.

7. Katz SL. Efficacy, potential and hazards of vaccines. *New England Journal of Medicine*. 1964;270(17):884–889.
8. Atchison RW, Casto BC, Hammon WM. Adenovirus-associated defective virus particles. *Science*. 1965;149(3685):754–756.
9. Hoggan MD, Blacklow NR, Rowe WP. Studies of small DNA viruses found in various adenovirus preparations: physical, biological, and immunological characteristics. *Proceedings of the National Academy of Sciences of the United States of America*. 1966;55(6):1467–1474.
10. Hastie E, Samulski RJ. Adeno-associated virus at 50: a golden anniversary of discovery, research, and gene therapy success—a personal perspective. *Human Gene Therapy*. 26(5):257–265.
11. Samulski RJ, Berns KI, Tan M, Muzyczka N. Cloning of adeno-associated virus into pBR322: rescue of intact virus from the recombinant plasmid in human cells. *Proceedings of the National Academy of Sciences of the United States of America*. 1982;79(6):2077–2081.
12. National Institutes of Health. Marshall Nirenberg: deciphering the genetic code—biographies. Office of NIH History and Stetten Museum. https://history.nih.gov/display/history/Nirenberg+Biographies/.
13. Ricki L. *The Forever Fix: Gene Therapy and the Boy Who Saved It*. St. Martin's; 2012.
14. Angier N. Girl, 4, becomes first human to receive engineered genes. *New York Times*. September 15, 1990. https://www.nytimes.com/1990/09/15/us/girl-4-becomes-first-human-to-receive-engineered-genes.html.
15. Mukherjee S. *The Gene: An Intimate History*. Scribner; 2016: 427–428.
16. Terry M. ABC's Robin Roberts kicks off BIO convention with keynote speech. BioSpace. June 5, 2018. https://www.biospace.com/article/abc-s-robin-roberts-kicks-off-bio-convention-with-keynote-speech/.
17. Stolberg SG. The biotech death of Jesse Gelsinger. *New York Times*. November 28, 1999. https://www.nytimes.com/1999/11/28/magazine/the-biotech-death-of-jesse-gelsinger.html.
18. Weiss TR, Nelson D. Teen dies undergoing experimental gene therapy. *Washington Post*. September 29, 1999. https://www.washingtonpost.com/wp-srv/WPcap/1999-09/29/060r-092999-idx.html.
19. Sibbald B. Death but one unintended consequence of gene-therapy trial. *Canadian Medical Association Journal*. 2001;164(11):1612.
20. Advisory Committee to the Director, Working Group on NIH Oversight of Clinical Gene Transfer Research. *Enhancing the Protection of Human Subjects in Gene Transfer Research at the National Institutes.*

National Institutes of Health. July 12, 2000. https://osp.od.nih.gov/wp-content/uploads/2014/03/acd_report_2000_07_12.pdf.

21. Wilson JM. Lessons learned from the gene therapy trial for ornithine transcarbamylase deficiency. *Molecular Genetics and Metabolism.* 2009; 96(4):151–157.

22. Rosenbaum L. Tragedy, perseverance, and chance—the story of CAR-T therapy. *New England Journal of Medicine.* 2017;377(14):1313–1315.

23. Bainbridge JW, Smith AJ, Barker SS, et al. Effect of gene therapy on visual function in Leber's congenital amaurosis. *New England Journal of Medicine.* 2008;358(21):2231–2239.

24. Cideciyan AV, Hauswirth WW, Aleman TS, et al. Human *RPE65* gene therapy for Leber congenital amaurosis: persistence of early visual improvements and safety at 1 year. *Human Gene Therapy.* 2009;20(9): 999–1004.

25. Maguire AM, Simonelli F, Pierce EA, et al. Safety and efficacy of gene transfer for Leber's congenital amaurosis. *New England Journal of Medicine.* 2008;358(21):2240–2248.

26. Rosner F. Hemophilia in the Talmud and rabbinic writings. *Annals of Internal Medicine.* 1969;70(4):833–837.

27. Stevens R. The history of haemophilia in the royal families of Europe. *British Journal of Haemotology.* 1999;105(1):25–32. https://online library.wiley.com/doi/10.1111/j.1365-2141.1999.01327.x/.

28. National Hemophilia Foundation. Hemophilia fast facts. https://www.hemophilia.org/About-Us/Fast-Facts/.

29. Biggs R, Douglas AS, MacFarlane RG, Dacie JV, Pitney WR. Christmas disease: a condition previously mistaken for haemophilia. *British Medical Journal.* 1952;2(4799):1378–1382.

30. Jones PK, Ratnoff OD. The changing prognosis of classic hemophilia (factor VIII "deficiency"). *Annals of Internal Medicine.* 1991;114(8): 641–648.

31. Darby SC, Kan SW, Spooner RJ, et al. Mortality rates, life expectancy, and causes of death in people with hemophilia A or B in the United Kingdom who were not infected with HIV. *Blood.* 2007;110(3):815–825.

32. Manco-Johnson MJ, Abshire TC, Shapiro AD, et al. Prophylaxis versus episodic treatment to prevent joint disease in boys with severe hemophilia. *New England Journal of Medicine.* 2007;357(6):535–544.

33. Nathwani AC, Tuddenham EG, Rangarajan S, et al. Adenovirus-associated virus vector-mediated gene transfer in hemophilia B. *New England Journal of Medicine.* 2011;365(25):2357–2365.

34. Nathwani AC, Reiss UM, Tuddenham EGD, et al. Long-term safety and efficacy of factor IX gene therapy in hemophilia B. *New England Journal of Medicine.* 2013;371(21):1994–2004.

35. European Medicines Agency. EPAR [European public assessment report] summary for the public: Glybera (alipogene tiparvovec). Last updated October 2015 [with the notation "Medicinal product no longer authorised"]. https://www.ema.europa.eu/docs/en_GB/document_library/EPAR_-_Summary_for_the_public/human/002145/WC500135474.pdf.

36. Sagonowsky E. With its launch fizzling out, UniQure gives up on $1M+ gene therapy Glybera. Fierce Pharma. April 20, 2017. https://www.fiercepharma.com/pharma/uniqure-gives-up-1m-gene-therapy-glybera/.

37. Moran N. First gene therapy approved. *Nature Biotechnology.* 2012; 30(12):1153. https://www.nature.com/articles/nbt1212-1153/.

38. Mijuk G. Novartis: breaking through barriers. Diversity Inc. November 27, 2018. https://www.diversityinc.com/novartis-breaking-through-barriers/.

39. Dominguez E, Marais T, Chatauret N, et al. Intravenous scAAV9 delivery of a codon-optimized *SMN1* sequence rescues SMA mice. *Human Molecular Genetics.* 2011;20(4):681–693. https://doi.org/10.1093/hmg/ddq514/.

40. Daya S, Berns KI. Gene therapy using adeno-associated virus vectors. *Clinical Microbiology Reviews.* 2008;21(4):583–593. https://www.ncbi.nlm.nih.gov/pmc/articles/PMC2570152/.

41. Apgar V. A proposal for a new method of evaluation of the newborn infant. *Current Researches in Anesthesia & Analgesia.* 1953;32(4):260–267.

chapter 5 **Sickle Cell Anemia**

1. Virginia Law. Description of the Virginia Sickle Cell Awareness Program. July 25, 2007. https://law.lis.virginia.gov/admincode/title12/agency5/chapter191/section290/.

2. Begley S. "Every time it's a battle": in excruciating pain, sickle cell patients are shunted aside. STAT News. September 18, 2017. https://www.statnews.com/2017/09/18/sickle-cell-pain-treatment/.

3. Lanzkron S , Carroll CP, Haywood C Jr. Mortality rates and age at death from sickle cell disease: U.S., 1979–2005. *Public Health Reports.* 2013; 128(2):110–116.

4. Lazio MP, Costello HH, Courtney DM, et al. A comparison of analgesic

management for emergency department patients with sickle cell disease and renal colic. *Clinical Journal of Pain.* 2010;26(3):199–205.

5. Savitt TL, Goldberg MF. Herrick's 1910 case report of sickle cell anemia: the rest of the story. *JAMA: Journal of the American Medical Association.* 1989;261(2):266–271.

6. Hahn EV, Gillespie EB. Report of a case greatly improved by splenectomy: experimental study of sickle cell formation. *Archives of Internal Medicine.* 1927;39(2):233–254.

7. Nobel Foundation. Linus Pauling: biographical. 1954. https://www.nobelprize.org/nobel_prizes/chemistry/laureates/1954/pauling-bio.html.

8. Linus Pauling Institute. Linus Pauling biography. Oregon State University. https://lpi.oregonstate.edu/about/linus-pauling-biography/.

9. Special Collections & Archives Resource Center (scarc). Pauling's theory of sickle cell anemia. December 11, 2008. The Pauling Blog. https://paulingblog.wordpress.com/2008/12/11/paulings-theory-of-sickle-cell-anemia/.

10. National Film Board of Canada. Pauling's interest in sickle cell anemia. Transcript of video clip from *Interview with Linus Pauling.* 1960. In: It's In the Blood! A Documentary History of Linus Pauling, Hemoglobin, and Sickle Cell Anemia. Special Collections & Archives Resource Center, Oregon State University. https://scarc.library.oregonstate.edu/coll/pauling/blood/video/1960v.34-interest.html.

11. Letter from Linus Pauling to William Castle. November 6, 1946. In: It's In the Blood! A Documentary History of Linus Pauling, Hemoglobin, and Sickle Cell Anemia. Special Collections & Archives Resource Center, Oregon State University. https://scarc.library.oregonstate.edu/coll/pauling/blood/corr/corr74.14-lp-castle-19461106.html.

12. Pauling L, Itano HA, Singer SJ, Wells IC. Sickle cell anemia, a molecular disease. *Science.* 1949;110(2865):543–548.

13. Allison AC. Protection afforded by sickle-cell trait against subtertian malariarial infection. *British Medical Journal.* 1954;1:290–294.

14. [Linus Pauling] narrative. Eugenics for alleviating human suffering. In: It's In the Blood! A Documentary History of Linus Pauling, Hemoglobin, and Sickle Cell Anemia; 35. Special Collections & Archives Resource Center, Oregon State University. https://scarc.library.oregonstate.edu/coll/pauling/blood/narrative/page35.html.

15. Special Collections & Archives Resource Center (scarc). Mastering genetics: Pauling and eugenics. February 24, 2009. The Pauling Blog.

https://paulingblog.wordpress.com/2009/02/24/mastering-genetics
-pauling-and-eugenics/.

16. Wailoo K. *Dying in the City of Blues: Sickle Cell Anemia and the Politics of Race and Health.* University of North Carolina Press; 2014: 165.

17. House steps up fight on sickle cell anemia. *Memphis Press-Scimitar.* October 8, 1971.

18. S[enate bill] 2676. A bill to provide for the prevention of sickle cell anemia. *Congressional Record—Senate,* vol. 117, pt. 27:S[enate]35596–35608. October 8, 1971. https://www.congress.gov/bound-congres sional-record/1971/10/08/senate-section/.

19. Nixon R. Statement on signing the National Sickle Cell Anemia Control Act. May 16, 1972. The American Presidency Project. https://www .presidency.ucsb.edu/documents/statement-signing-the-national-sickle -cell-anemia-control-act/.

20. Charache S, Dover G, Smith K, Talbot CC Jr, Moyer M, Boyer S. Treatment of sickle cell anemia with 5-azacytidine results in increased fetal hemoglobin production and is associated with nonrandom hypomethylation of DNA around the γ-δ-β globin gene complex. *Proceedings of the National Academy of Sciences of the United States of America.* 1983; 80(15):4842–4846.

21. Switched-on genes. *Newsweek.* December 20, 1982; 85.

22. Cisneros GS, Thein SL. Recent advances in the treatment of sickle cell disease. *Frontiers in Physiology.* 2020;11:435. https://www.frontiersin .org/articles/10.3389/fphys.2020.00435/full/.

23. Rodgers GP, Dover GJ, Noguchi CT, Schechter AN, Nienhuis AW. Hematologic responses of patients with sickle cell disease to treatment with hydroxyurea. *New England Journal of Medicine.* 1990;322(15):1037–1045.

24. Leary WE. Drug is promising in sickle-cell test. *New York Times.* April 12, 1990. https://www.nytimes.com/1990/04/12/us/drug-is-promis ing-in-sickle-cell-test.html.

25. Charache S, Terrin ML, Moore RD, et al. Effect of hydroxyurea on the frequency of painful crises in sickle cell anemia. *New England Journal of Medicine.* 1995;332(20):1317–1322.

26. Ho PTC, Murgo AJ. Hydroxyurea and sickle cell crisis. *New England Journal of Medicine.* 1995;333(15):1008–1009.

27. Droxia® (hydroxyurea capsules, USP). Bristol-Myers Squibb. March 4, 1998; revised January 2012. https://www.accessdata.fda.gov/drugsatfda _docs/label/2012/016295s041s042lbl.pdf.

28. US Food and Drug Administration news release. FDA approves new treatment for sickle cell disease. July 7, 2017. https://www.fda.gov/news -events/press-announcements/fda-approves-new-treatment-sickle -cell-disease/.

29. US Food and Drug Administration news release. FDA approves first targeted therapy to treat patients with painful complication of sickle cell disease. November 15, 2019. https://www.fda.gov/news-events /press-announcements/fda-approves-first-targeted-therapy-treat -patients-painful-complication-sickle-cell-disease/.

30. US Food and Drug Administration. FDA approves new voxelotor for sickle cell disease. November 25, 2019. https://www.fda.gov/drugs /resources-information-approved-drugs/fda-approves-voxelotor-sickle -cell-disease/.

chapter 6 *Ex Vivo* Gene Therapy

1. National Heart, Lung, and Blood Institute. Fanconi amemia. https:// www.nhlbi.nih.gov/health-topics/fanconi-anemia/.

2. Cavazzana-Calvo M, Hacein-Bey S, de Saint Basile G, et al. Gene therapy of human severe combined immunodeficiency (SCID)-X1 disease. *Science*. 2000;288(5466):669–672.

3. Anderson WF. The best of times, the worst of times. *Science*. 2000;288 (5466):627–629.

4. Hacein-Bey-Abina S, Le Deist F, Carlier F, et al. Sustained correction of X-linked severe combined immunodeficiency by *ex vivo* gene therapy. *New England Journal of Medicine*. 2002;346(16):1185–1193.

5. Cavazzana M, Six E, Lagresle-Peyrou C, Andre-Schmutz I, Hacein-Bey-Abina S. Gene therapy for X-linked severe combined immunodeficiency: where do we stand? *Human Gene Therapy*. 2016;27(2):108–116. https://doi.org/10.1089/hum.2015.137/.

6. Markwick C. FDA halts gene therapy trials after leukaemia case in France. *British Medical Journal*. 2003;326(7382):181. Also see Mcdowell N. New cancer case halts US gene therapy trials. *New Scientist*. January 15, 2003.

7. Cavazzana-Calvo M, Payen E, Negre O, et al. Transfusion independence and *HMGA2* activation after gene therapy of human β-thalassemia. *Nature*. 2010;467(7313):318–322.

8. bluebird bio press release. NATURE publishes promising results on treatment of first patient in bluebird bio's Phase 1/2 beta-thalassemia study.

September 15, 2010. https://investor.bluebirdbio.com/news-releases/news-release-details/nature-publishes-promising-results-treatment-first-patient/.

9. Pawliuk R, Westerman KA, Fabry ME, et al. Correction of sickle cell disease in transgenic mouse models by gene therapy. *Science*. 2001;294 (5550):2368–2371.

10. Ribeil JA, Hacein-Bey-Abina S, Payen E, et al. Gene therapy in a patient with sickle cell disease. *New England Journal of Medicine*. 2017;376(9): 848–855.

11. ClinicalTrials.gov. A study evaluating the safety and efficacy of bb1111 in severe sickle cell disease. May 16, 2014. https://clinicaltrials.gov/ct2/show/NCT02140554?term=LentiGLobin+sickle+cell&rank=1/.

12. Pinto D. Gene therapy LentiGlobin continues to show good results, bluebird bio says. Sickle Cell Disease News. June 28, 2018. https://sicklecellanemianews.com/2018/06/28/gene-therapy-lentiglobin-continues-show-good-results-study/.

13. bluebird bio press release. New data show near elimination of sickle cell disease–related vaso-occlusive crises and acute chest syndrome in Phase 1/2 clinical study of bluebird bio's LentiGlobin™ gene therapy for sickle cell disease at 25th EHA Congress. June 12, 2020. https://investor.bluebirdbio.com/news-releases/news-release-details/new-data-show-near-elimination-sickle-cell-disease-related-vaso/.

14. bluebird bio press release. bluebird bio provides updated findings from reported case of acute myeloid leukemia (AML) in LentiGlobin for sickle cell disease (SCD) gene therapy program. March 10, 2021. https://investor.bluebirdbio.com/news-releases/news-release-details/bluebird-bio-provides-updated-findings-reported-case-acute/.

15. Kolata G. These patients had sickle-cell disease: experimental therapies might have cured them. *New York Times*. January 27, 2019. https://www.nytimes.com/2019/01/27/health/sickle-cell-gene-therapy.html.

16. Ishino Y, Shinagawa H, Makino K, Amemura M, Nakata A. Nucleotide sequence of the iap gene, responsible for alkaline phosphatase isozyme conversion in *Escherichia coli*, and the identification of the gene product. *Journal of Bacteriology*. 1987;169(12):5429–5433.

17. *Nature Medicine* editorial. Keep off-target effects in focus. *Nature Medicine*. 2018;24:1081. https://www.nature.com/articles/s41591-018-0150-3/.

18. Barrangou R, Fremaux C, Deveau H, et al. CRISPR provides acquired resistance against viruses in prokaryotes. *Science*. 2007;315(5819):1709–1712.

19. Jinek M, Chylinski K, Fonfara I, Hauer M, Doudna JA, Charpentier E. A programmable dual-RNA-guided DNA endonuclease in adaptive bacterial immunity. *Science*. 2012;337(6096):816–821.

20. Cong L, Ran FA, Dox D, et al. Multiplex genome engineering using CRISPR/Cas systems. *Science*. 2013;339(6121):819–823.

21. Plummer B, Barclay E, Bellz J, Irfan U. A simple guide to CRISPR, one of the biggest science stories of the decade. Vox. Updated December 27, 2018. https://www.vox.com/2018/7/23/17594864/crispr-cas9-gene -editing/.

22. Peyton B, director. *Rampage*. Warner Bros. 2018.

23. Doudna JA, Sternberg SH. *A Crack in Creation: Gene Editing and the Unthinkable Power to Control Evolution*. Houghton Mifflin Harcourt; 2017.

24. Stein R. The CRISPR revolution: a young Mississippi woman's journey through a pioneering gene-editing experiment. Shots: Health News from NPR. December 25, 2019. https://www.npr.org/sections/health -shots/2019/12/25/784395525/a-young-mississippi-womans-journey -through-a-pioneering-gene-editing-experiment/.

25. Frangoul H, Bobruff Y, Cappellini MD, et al. Safety and efficacy of CTX001 in patients with transfusion-dependent β-thalassemia and sickle cell disease: early results from the CLIMB THAL-111 and CLIMB SCD-121 studies of autologous CRISPR-CAS9–modified CD34+ hematopoietic stem and progenitor cells. Paper presented at: 62nd ASH Annual Meeting and Exposition, a Virtual Experience, December 5–8, 2020. American Society of Hematology. https://ash.confex.com/ash /2020/webprogram/Paper139575.html.

26. Grupp S, Bloberger N, Campbell C, et al. CTX001™ for sickle cell disease: safety and efficacy results from the ongoing CLIMB SCD-121 study of autologous CRISPR-Cas9-modified CD34+ hematopoietic stem and progenitor cells. PowerPoint presentation at: EHA 2021, Virtual, June 9–17, 2021. European Hematology Association. https://ir .crisprtx.com/static-files/1db0ff23-41dd-4f1a-a523-456ecf7991b8/.

chapter 7 A Brief History of FDA Regulations

1. Constitutional Rights Foundation. Upton Sinclair's *The Jungle*: muckraking the meat-packing industry. Bill of Rights in Action. https://www .crf-usa.org/bill-of-rights-in-action/bria-24-1-b-upton-sinclairs-the -jungle-muckraking-the-meat-packing-industry.html.

2. US Food and Drug Administration. FDA history research tools. https:// www.fda.gov/about-fda/fda-history/fda-history-research-tools/.

3. Cavers DF. The Food, Drug, and Cosmetic Act of 1938: its legislative history and its substantive provisions. *Law and Contemporary Problems*. 1939;6(1):1–42. https://scholarship.law.duke.edu/cgi/viewcontent.cgi ?article=1937&context=lcp/.

4. Roosevelt FD. Special message to the Congress of the United States. *Congressional Record—Senate*, vol. 79, pt. 4:S[enate]4262. March 22, 1935. https://www.congress.gov/bound-congressional-record/1935/03 /22/senate-section/.

5. *Life* on the American newsfront: bad medicine leaves trail of dead patients. *Life*. November 8, 1937. The photo of Dr. Archie Calhoun, shown examining a bottle of elixir of sulfanilamide, is reproduced in Yuzuki D. The origin of the FDA and the elixir sulfanilamide disaster of 1937. Singtlera Genomics. March 19, 2019. https://singleraoncology.com/the -origin-of-the-fda-and-the-elixir-sulfanilamide-disaster-of-1937/.

6. Ballentine C. Taste of rasberries, taste of death: the 1937 elixir sulfanilamide incident. *FDA Consumer Magazine*. June 1981. https://www.gmp trainingsystems.com/files/u1/pdf/Sulfanilamide_article.pdf.

7. Lesser W. *American Business Regulation: Understand, Survive, and Thrive*. Taylor & Francis; 2015.

8. Eriksson T, Bjorkman S, Hoglund P. Clinical pharmacology of thalidomide. *Eurupean Journal of Clinical Pharmacology*. 2001;57(5):365–376.

9. Evans H. Thalidomide: how men who blighted lives of thousands evaded justice. *Guardian* (Manchester). November 14, 2014. https://www.the guardian.com/society/2014/nov/14/-sp-thalidomide-pill-how-evaded -justice/.

10. McBride WG. Letter to the editor: thalidomide and congenital abnormalities. *Lancet*. 1961;278(7216):1358.

11. Lenz W. The history of thalidomide. Lecture given at: UNITH [United International Thalidomides = International Thalidomide Society] Congress. 1992. https://www.thalidomide.ca/wp-content/uploads/2017 /12/Dr-Lenz-history-of-thalidomide-1992.pdf.

12. Dove F. What's happened to thalidomide babies? BBC News. November 3, 2011. https://www.bbc.com/news/magazine-15536544/.

13. Tantibanchachai C. U.S. regulatory response to thalidomide (1950–2000). The Embryo Project Encyclopedia. April 1, 2014. https://embryo .asu.edu/pages/us-regulatory-response-thalidomide-1950-2000/.

14. Taussig HB. The thalidomide syndrome. *Scientific American*. 1962;207 (2):29–35.
15. HIV.gov. A timeline of HIV and AIDS. https://www.aids.gov/hiv-basics /overview/history/hiv-and-aids-timeline/.
16. Haverkos HW, Curran JW. The current outbreak of Kaposi's sarcoma and opportunistic infections. *CA: A Cancer Journal for Clinicians*. 1982; 32(6):330–338.
17. Carpenter D. *Reputation and Power: Organizational Image and Pharmaceutical Regulation at the FDA*. Princeton University Press; 2014.
18. Crimp D. Before Occupy: how AIDS activists seized control of the FDA in 1988. *Atlantic*. December 6, 2011. https://www.theatlantic.com /health/archive/2011/12/before-occupy-how-aids-activists-seized -control-of-the-fda-in-1988/249302/.
19. US Food and Drug Administration. Accelerated approval. January 4, 2018. https://www.fda.gov/patients/fast-track-breakthrough-therapy -accelerated-approval-priority-review/accelerated-approval/.
20. See Applications for FDA approval to market a new drug: approval with restrictions to assure safe use. *Code of Federal Regulations*. 2021; Title 21:314.520. Also see Licensing: approval with restrictions to assure safe use. *Code of Federal Regulations*. 2021;Title 21:601.42. Both are available at https://www.accessdata.fda.gov/scripts/cdrh/cfdocs /cfcfr/cfrsearch.cfm.
21. Cohen M, Johnson JR, Pazdur R. U.S. Food and Drug Administration drug approval summary: conversion of imatinib mesylate (STI571; Gleevec) tablets from accelerated approval to full approval. *Clinical Cancer Research*. 2005;11(1):12–19. https://pubmed.ncbi.nlm.nih.gov /15671523/#:~:text=After%202%20years%20of%20treatment,inter val%2C%2088.3%2D93.2)/.
22. Feuerstein A, Harper M, Garde D. Inside "Project Onyx": how Biogen used an FDA back channel to win approval of its polarizing Alzheimer's drug. MSN News. June 29, 2021. https://www.msn.com/en-us/news/us /inside-project-onyx-how-biogen-used-an-fda-back-channel-to-win-ap proval-of-its-polarizing-alzheimers-drug/ar-AALzzpL/.
23. Alexander RC, Knopman DS, Emerson SS, et al. Revisiting FDA approval of Aducanumab. *New England Journal of Medicine*. 2021;385(9): 769–771. https://www.nejm.org/doi/full/10.1056/NEJMp2110468/.
24. Office of the Inspector General. Review of the FDA's accelerated approval pathway. US Department of Health and Human Services.

https://oig.hhs.gov/reports-and-publications/workplan/summary/wp
-summary-0000608.asp.

25. US Food and Drug Administration. Prescription Drug User Fee Amendments. https://www.fda.gov/industry/fda-user-fee-programs/prescription-drug-user-fee-amendments/.

26. US Food and Drug Administration. Food and Drug Administration Safety and Innovation Act (FDASIA). https://www.fda.gov/regulatory-information/selected-amendments-fdc-act/food-and-drug-administration-safety-and-innovation-act-fdasia/.

27. Dabrowska A, Thaul S. *Prescription Drug User Fee Act (PDUFA): 2017 Reauthorization as PDUFA VI*. Congressional Research Service. March 16, 2018. https://fas.org/sgp/crs/misc/R44864.pdf.

chapter 8 **The Path to Approval**

1. US Food and Drug Administration. What is an FDA Advisory Committee? https://www.fda.gov/about-fda/fda-basics/what-fda-advisory-committee/.

2. US Food and Drug Administration. Committees and meeting materials. https://www.fda.gov/advisory-committees/committees-and-meeting-materials/.

3. US Food and Drug Administration. 2017 meeting materials: Oncologic Drugs Advisory Committee. July 12, 2017. https://www.fda.gov/advisory-committees/oncologic-drugs-advisory-committee/2017-meeting-materials-oncologic-drugs-advisory-committee/.

4. Feuerstein A, Garde D. Novel gene therapy for leukemia clears FDA panel. STAT News. July 13, 2017. https://www.scientificamerican.com/article/novel-gene-therapy-for-leukemia-clears-fda-panel/.

5. Whitehead E. Carl June. *Time*. 2018. https://time.com/collection/most-influential-people-2018/5238121/carl-june/.

6. US Food and Drug Administration news release. FDA approval brings first gene therapy to the United States. August 30, 2017. https://www.fda.gov/news-events/press-announcements/fda-approval-brings-first-gene-therapy-united-states/.

7. Gilead press release. Kite Pharma announces positive topline KTE-C19 data from ZUMA-1 pivotal trial in patients with aggressive non-Hodgkin lymphoma (NHL). September 26, 2016. https://www.gilead.com/news-and-press/press-room/press-releases/2016/9/kite-pharma-announces

-positive-topline-ktec19-data-from-zuma1-pivotal-trial-in-patients-with
-aggressive-nonhodgkin-lymphoma-nhl/.

8. Havert M, chair of review committee. Summary basis for regulatory action: YESCARTA™ (axicabtagene ciloleucel). October 18, 2017. https://www.fda.gov/media/108788/download/.

9. Urban R. JPM at 15. Johnson & Johnson Innovation. January 4, 2018. https://jnjinnovation.com/node/blog-post/jpm-15/.

10. J.P. Morgan 40th Annual Healthcare Conference (#JPM2022)—now VIRTUAL! Digital Health Today. January 2022. https://digitalhealthtoday.com/events/jp-morgan-global-healthcare-conference/#:~:text=What%20is%20today%20known%20as,Hambrecht%20%26%20Quist%20(H%26Q).&text=At%20its%20infancy%2C%20the%20conference,still%20at%20the%20Westin%20St/.

11. US Securities and Exchange Commission. Schedule 14D-9: Kite Pharma, Inc. https://www.sec.gov/Archives/edgar/data/1510580/000119312517276737/d450961dsc14d9.htm.

12. Kim T. Goldman Sachs asks in biotech research report: "Is curing patients a sustainable business model?" CNBC. April 11, 2018. https://www.cnbc.com/2018/04/11/goldman-asks-is-curing-patients-a-sustainable-business-model.html.

13. Gilead press release. Gilead Sciences to acquire Kite Pharma for $11.9 billion. August 28, 2017. https://www.gilead.com/news/press-releases/2017/8/gilead-sciences-to-acquire-kite-pharma-for-119-billion/.

14. Gilead press release. Kite's Yescarta™ (axicabtagene ciloleucel) becomes first CAR T therapy approved by the FDA for the treatment of adult patients with relapsed or refractory large B-cell lymphoma after two or more lines of systemic therapy. October 18, 2018. https://www.gilead.com/news-and-press/press-room/press-releases/2017/10/kites-yescarta-axicabtagene-ciloleucel-becomes-first-car-t-therapy-approved-by-the-fda-for-the-treatment-of-adult-patients-with-relapsed-or-refrac/.

15. Life Sci VC blog. Two CARTs, two charts: dissecting returns from T-cell therapy M&A. January 23, 2018. https://lifescivc.com/2018/01/two-carts-two-charts-dissecting-returns-t-cell-therapy-ma/.

16. Lovelace B Jr. Juno Therapeutics shares plunge after FDA place clinical hold on cancer trial. CNBC. July 8, 2016. https://www.cnbc.com/2016/07/08/juno-therapeutics-shares-plunge-after-fda-place-clinical-hold-on-cancer-trial.html.

17. Clinical holds and requests for modification. *Code of Federal Regula-*

tions. 2021;Title 21:312.42. https://www.accessdata.fda.gov/scripts
/cdrh/cfdocs/cfcfr/CFRSearch.cfm?fr=312.42/.
18. Mangan D, Tirrell M. Juno Therapeutics shares soar as clinical trial re-
sumes. CNBC. July 12, 2016. https://www.cnbc.com/2016/07/12/juno
-therapeutics-shares-soar-as-clinical-hold-removed.html.
19. Broderick JM. Clinical hold again placed on Phase II trial of JCAR015 in
ALL. OncLive. November 23, 2016. https://www.onclive.com/web-ex
clusives/clinical-hold-again-placed-on-phase-ii-trial-of-jcar015-in-all/.
20. Couzin-Frankel J. Worries, confusion after cancer trial deaths. *Science.*
2016;354(6317):1211. https://science.sciencemag.org/content/354
/6317/1211/.
21. Center for Responsible Science. Watchdog group files amendment to
FDA citizen petition after 20 deaths in clinical drug trials. Pharmaceutical Processing World. May 17, 2017. https://www.pharmpro.com/news
/2017/05/watchdog-group-files-amendment-fda-citizen-petition-after
-20-deaths-clinical-drug-trials/.
22. Lash A. After trial deaths, Juno pivots and scraps lead CAR-T therapy.
Xconomy. March 1, 2017. https://www.xconomy.com/seattle/2017/03
/01/after-trial-deaths-juno-pivots-and-scraps-lead-car-t-therapy/.
23. Dangler R. Cancer immunotherapy company tries to explain deaths in
recent trial. Science Insider. November 16, 2017. https://www.science
.org/content/article/cancer-immunotherapy-company-tries-explain
-deaths-recent-trial/. Also see News in Brief. JCAR015 in ALL: a root-
cause investigation. *Cancer Discovery.* 2018;8(1):4–5. https://cancerdis
covery.aacrjournals.org/content/8/1/4.3/.
24. News in Brief. JCAR015 in ALL: a root-cause investigation. *Cancer Discovery.* 2018;8(1):4–5. https://cancerdiscovery.aacrjournals.org/content
/8/1/4.3/.
25. US Food and Drug Administration news release. FDA approves new
treatment for adults with relapsed or refractory large-B-cell lymphoma,
February 5, 2021. https://www.fda.gov/news-events/press-announce
ments/fda-approves-new-treatment-adults-relapsed-or-refractory-large
-b-cell-lymphoma/.
26. US Securities and Exchange Commission. Schedule 14D-9 filing: Juno
Therapeutics, Inc. https://www.sec.gov/Archives/edgar/data/1594864
/000119312518030824/d514862dsc14d9.htm.
27. Celgene press release. Celgene Corporation to acquire Juno Therapeutics, Inc., advancing global leadership in cellular immunotherapy. Janu-

ary 22, 2018. https://ir.celgene.com//press-releases-archive/press-re lease-details/2018/Celgene-Corporation-to-Acquire-Juno-Therapeutics -Inc-Advancing-Global-Leadership-in-Cellular-Immunotherapy/de fault.aspx.

28. Russell S, Bennett J, Wellman JA, et al. Efficacy and safety of voretigene neparvovec (AAV2-hRPE65v2) in patients with *RPE65*-mediated in- herited retinal dystrophy: a randomised, controlled, open-label, phase 3 trial. *Lancet*. 2017;390(10097):849–6860.

29. US Food and Drug Administration. Spark Therapeutic, Inc.—Voretigene neparvovec (AAV2-hRPE65v2): draft discussion questions (clinical) for the [Cellular, Tissue, and Gene Therapies] Advisory Committee (AC). October 12, 2017. https://www.fda.gov/media/108205/download/.

30. US Food and Drug Administration. 67th Meeting of the Cellular, Tissue, and Gene Therapies Advisory Committee. October 12, 2017. https:// www.fda.gov/media/109384/download/.

31. US Food and Drug Administration news release. FDA approves novel gene therapy to treat patients with a rare form of inherited vision loss. December 18, 2017. https://www.fda.gov/news-events/press-an nouncements/fda-approves-novel-gene-therapy-treat-patients-rare -form-inherited-vision-loss/.

32. Mass[achusetts] Eye and Ear Communications. Making gene therapy history. April 2, 2018. https://focus.masseyeandear.org/making-gene -therapy-history/.

33. Mass[achusetts] Eye and Ear Communications. Two months after gene therapy, Jack sees brighter, more clearly. May 22, 2018. https://focus .masseyeandear.org/two-months-after-gene-therapy-jack-sees-a-little -brighter-more-clearly/.

34. Kegel M. Updates from trial of AveXis *SMA1* gene therapy trial show impressive results in most infants. SMA News Today. April 25, 2017. https://smanewstoday.com/news-posts/2017/04/25/sma1-gene-ther apy-avxs-101-infants-clinical-trial/. Also see Dotinga R. Gene therapy for spinal muscular atrophy shows promise in early study. MDedge/ Neurology. July 1, 2017. https://www.mdedge.com/clinicalneurology news/article/141703/pediatrics/gene-therapy-spinal-muscular-atro phy-shows-promise/.

35. Mendell JR, Al-Zaidy S, Shell R, et al. Single-dose gene-replacement therapy for spinal muscular atrophy. *New England Journal of Medicine*. 2017;377(18):1713–1722.

36. Collins F. Clinical trials bring hope to kids with spinal muscular atrophy. NIH Director's Blog. November 21, 2017. https://directorsblog.nih.gov/2017/11/21/clinical-trials-bring-hope-to-kids-with-spinal-muscular-atrophy/.

37. US Securities and Exchange Commission. Schedule 14D-9 filing: AveXis Inc. April 17, 2018. https://www.sec.gov/Archives/edgar/data/1652923/000104746918002890/a2235337zsc14d9.htm.

38. Novartis press release. Novartis enters agreement to acquire AveXis Inc. for USD 8.7 b[illio]n to transform care in SMA and expand position as a gene therapy and neuroscience leader. April 9, 2018. https://www.novartis.com/news/media-releases/novartis-enters-agreement-acquire-avexis-inc-usd-87-bn-transform-care-sma-and-expand-position-gene-therapy-and-neuroscience-leader/.

39. Novartis press release. AveXis receives FDA approval for Zolgensma®, the first and only gene therapy for pediatric patients with spinal muscular atrophy (SMA). May 24, 2019. https://www.novartis.com/news/media-releases/avexis-receives-fda-approval-zolgensma-first-and-only-gene-therapy-pediatric-patients-spinal-muscular-atrophy-sma/.

40. Feuerstein A. Novartis was aware of manipulation of data supporting gene therapy approval, FDA says. STAT News. August 6, 2019. https://www.statnews.com/2019/08/06/novartis-was-aware-of-manipulation-of-data-supporting-gene-therapy-approval-fda-says/.

41. US Food and Drug Administration statement. Statement on data accuracy issues with recently approved gene therapy. https://www.fda.gov/news-events/press-announcements/statement-data-accuracy-issues-recently-approved-gene-therapy/.

42. Califf RM. Novartis violated FDA's sacred principle: in God we trust, all others must bring data. STAT News. August 14, 2019. https://www.statnews.com/2019/08/14/fda-novartis-zolgensma-data-integrity/?utm_content=bufferdfa1f&utm_medium=social&utm_source=twitter&utm_campaign=twitter_organic/.

43. Reuters. FDA takes no action against Novartis after gene therapy data inquiry. Yahoo/News. March 31, 2020. https://news.yahoo.com/fda-takes-no-action-against-174225768.html.

44. US Food and Drug Administration. The voice of the patient: sickle cell disease. October 2014. https://www.fda.gov/media/89898/download/.

45. Stein R. The CRISPR Revolution: in a 1st, doctors in U.S. use CRISPR tool to treat patient with genetic disorder. Shots: Health News from NPR.

July 29, 2019. https://www.npr.org/sections/health-shots/2019/07/29 /744826505/sickle-cell-patient-reveals-why-she-is-volunteering-for -landmark-gene-editing-st/.

46. National Institutes of Health news release. NIH launches initiative to accelerate genetic therapies to cure sickle cell disease. National Institutes of Health. September 13, 2018. https://www.nih.gov/news-events/news -releases/nih-launches-initiative-accelerate-genetic-therapies-cure -sickle-cell-disease/.

47. American Society of Hematology press release. ASH president: NIH Cure Sickle Cell Initiative "bold and visionary." American Society of Hematology. September 13, 2018. https://www.hematology.org/newsroom/press -releases/2018/nih-cure-sickle-cell-initiative-bold-visionary/.

48. Adair JE, Androski L, Bayigga L, et al. Towards access for all: 1st Working Group Report for the Global Gene Therapy Initiative (GGTI). *Gene Therapy.* 2021;September 8. https://www.nature.com/articles/s41434 -021-00284-4/.

49. McCune JM, Stevenson SC, Doehle BP, Trenor CC III, Turner EH, Spector JM. Collaborative science to advance gene therapies in resource-limited parts of the world. *Molecular Therapy.* 2010;29(11):3101-31012. https://doi.org/10.1016/j.ymthe.2021.05.024/.

chapter 9 **Building Blocks**

1. Dunbar CE, High KA, Joung JK, Kohn DB, Ozawa K, Sadelain M.. Gene therapy comes of age. *Science.* 2018;359(6372): 175.

2. Grant AM. *Originals: How Non-Conformists Change the World.* Penguin Books; 2017.

3. Isaacson W. *Leonardo da Vinci: A New Biography.* Simon & Schuster; 2017.

4. Afeyan N, Pisano GP. What evolution can teach us about innovation. *Harvard Business Review.* September/October 2021. https://hbr.org /2021/09/what-evolution-can-teach-us-about-innovation/.

5. Tversky A, Kahneman D. Advances in prospect theory: cumulative representation of uncertainty. *Journal of Risk and Uncertainty.* 1992;5(4): 297–323. https://link.springer.com/article/10.1007%2FBF00122574/.

6. Staats BR. *Never Stop Learning: Stay Relevant, Reinvent Yourself, and Thrive.* Harvard Business Review Press; 2018.

7. Heider F. *The Psychology of Interpersonal Relations.* Wiley; 1958.

8. Gladwell M. *The Tipping Point: How Little Things Make a Big Difference.* Little, Brown; 2011.

9. Jones BF, Weinberg BA. Age dynamics in scientific creativity. *Proceedings of the National Academy of Sciences of the United States of America.* 2011;108(47):18910–18914.

10. Weinberg BA, Galenson DW. Creative careers: the life cycles of Nobel laureates in economics. November 2005; revised November 2007. NBER [National Bureau of Economic Research] Working Paper No. 11799. https://www.nber.org/papers/w11799/.

11. Kneller R. The importance of new companies for drug discovery: origins of a decade of new drugs. *Nature Reviews Drug Discovery.* 2010;9(12): 867–883.

12. Wu L, Wang D, Evans JA. Large teams develop and small teams disrupt science and technology. *Nature.* 2019;566(7744):378–382. https://doi .org/10.1038/s41586-019-0941-9/.

13. Poteyeva M. Social capital. *Encyclopedia Brittanica* online. https://www .britannica.com/topic/social-capital/.

chapter 10 **Recognizing Value**

1. Transcript from Martin Shkreli congressional hearing, House Committee on Oversight and Government Reform. February 4, 2016. CNN Transcripts. February 4, 2016. http://www.cnn.com/TRANSCRIPTS /1602/04/qmb.01.html.

2. Ayres C. Martin Shkreli: the most hated millennial in America. *GQ.* January 3, 2017. https://www.gq-magazine.co.uk/article/martin -shkreli/.

3. Abdullah H. 'Pharma bro' Shkreli invokes the Fifth before Congress. NBC News. Updated February 4, 2016. https://www.nbcnews.com/news/us -news/pharma-bro-martin-shkreli-faces-congress-n511106/.

4. McGinley L. Childhood cancer survivors face "financial toxicity." *Washington Post.* August 1, 2018. https://www.washingtonpost.com/news/to -your-health/wp/2018/08/01/childhood-cancer-survivors-face-finan cial-toxicity/?noredirect=on&utm_term=.689143d9dbf0/.

5. Thomas K, Ornstein C. The price they pay. *New York Times.* March 5, 2018. https://www.nytimes.com/2018/03/05/health/drug-prices.html.

6. National Cancer Institute. Financial toxicity. https://www.cancer.gov/ publications/dictionaries/cancer-terms/def/financial-toxicity/.

7. Kaiser Family Foundation. Retail prescription drugs filled at pharmacies per capita. 2019. https://www.kff.org/health-costs/state-indicator/retail-rx-drugs-per-capita/?currentTimeframe=0&selectedDistributions=retail-rx-drugs-per-capita&selectedRows=%7B%22wrapups%22:%7B%22united-states%22:%7B%7D%7D%7D&sortModel=%7B%22colId%22:%22Retail%20Rx%20Drugs%20per%20Capita%22,%22sort%22:%22desc%22%7D/.

8. Huang I-C, Bhakta N, Brinkman TM, et al. Determinants and consequences of financial hardship among adult survivors of childhood cancer: a report from the St. Jude lifetime cohort study. *JNCI: Journal of the National Cancer Institute.* 2019;111(2):189–200. https://doi.org/10.1093/jnci/djy120/.

9. Centers for Disease Control and Prevention. *Health, United States, 2016, with Chartbook on Long-Term Trends in Health.* US Department of Health and Human Services. May 2017. https://www.cdc.gov/nchs/data/hus/hus16.pdf.

10. Fein AJ. Tales of the unsurprised: brand-name drug prices fell for the fourth consecutive year. Drug Channels. January 4, 2022. https://www.drugchannels.net/2022/01/tales-of-unsurprised-brand-name-drug.html.

11. Dave CV, Hartzema A, Kesselheim AS. Prices of generic drugs associated with numbers of manufacturers. *New England Journal of Medicine.* 2017;377(26)2597–2598. https://www.nejm.org/doi/full/10.1056/NEJMc1711899/.

12. LaMattina J. When it comes to abusive drug pricing, don't confuse Shkreli with hep C drugs. *Forbes.* July 19, 2017. https://www.forbes.com/sites/johnlamattina/2017/07/19/when-it-comes-to-abusive-drug-pricing-dont-confuse-shkreli-with-hep-c-drugs/.

13. Centers for Disease Control and Prevention. Viral hepatitis: Q&As for the public. July 28, 2020. https://www.cdc.gov/hepatitis/hcv/cfaq.htm.

14. Gilead press release. U.S. Food and Drug Administration approves Gilead's Sovaldi™ (sofosbuvir) for the treatment of chronic hepatitis C. December 6, 2016. https://www.gilead.com/news-and-press/press-room/press-releases/2013/12/us-food-and-drug-administration-approves-gileads-sovaldi-sofosbuvir-for-the-treatment-of-chronic-hepatitis-c/.

15. Pollack A. Harvoni, a hepatitis C drug from Gilead, wins FDA approval. *New York Times.* October 11, 2014. https://www.nytimes.com/2014/10/11/business/harvoni-a-hepatitis-c-drug-from-gilead-wins-fda-approval.html.

16. Bach PB, Trusheim M. The U.S. government should buy Gilead for $156 billion to save money on hepatitis C. *Forbes*. January 17, 2017. https://www.forbes.com/sites/sciencebiz/2017/01/17/the-u-s-government-should-buy-gilead-for-156-billion-to-save-money-on-hepatitis-c/#2cd0490c71a2/.

17. Johnson CY. Louisiana adopts "Netflix" model to pay for hepatitis C drugs. *Washington Post*. January 10, 2019. https://www.washingtonpost.com/health/2019/01/10/louisiana-adopts-netflix-model-pay-hepatitis-c-drugs/?noredirect=on&utm_term=.1f1ed34ed7b1/.

18. Life Sci VC blog. Innovators vs exploiters: drug pricing and the future of pharma. August 29, 2016. https://lifescivc.com/2016/08/innovators-vs-exploiters-drug-pricing-future-pharma/.

19. Parsa-Parsi RW. The revised Declaration of Geneva: a modern-day physician's pledge. *JAMA: Journal of the American Medical Association*. 2017;318(2):1971–1972.

20. More B. Drug executives should take a Hippocratic oath. *Nature*. 2018;555(7698):561.

21. Fox E. How pharma companies game the system to keep drugs expensive. *Harvard Business Review*. April 6, 2017. https://hbr.org/2017/04/how-pharma-companies-game-the-system-to-keep-drugs-expensive/.

22. Merck GW. Speech delivered at the Medical College of Virginia. 1950. https://www.merck.com/company-overview/history/.

23. Rockoff JD. The million-dollar cancer treatment: who will pay? *Wall Street Journal*. April 26, 2018. https://www.wsj.com/articles/the-million-dollar-cancer-treatment-no-one-knows-how-to-pay-for-1524740401/.

24. Pearl R. Healthcare's dangerous fee-for-service addiction. *Forbes*. September 25, 2017. https://www.forbes.com/sites/robertpearl/2017/09/25/fee-for-service-addiction/#5cfd58bbc8ad/.

25. Rosenberg CE. *The Care of Strangers: The Rise of America's Hospital System*. Basic Books; 1987.

26. Blue Cross and Blue Shield. Health insurance from invention to innovation: a history of the Blue Cross and Blue Shield companies. November 11, 2012. https://www.bcbs.com/articles/health-insurance-invention-innovation-history-of-the-blue-cross-and-blue-shield/. Also see Blue Cross and Blue Shield. Blue Cross: origins. https://www.bcbs.com/about-us/industry-pioneer/.

27. Chatterjee A, Dougan C, Tevelow BJ, Zamani A. Innovative pharma contracts: when do value-based arrangements work? McKinsey &

Company. October 19, 2017. https://www.mckinsey.com/industries /pharmaceuticals-and-medical-products/our-insights/innovative -pharma-contracts-when-do-value-based-arrangements-work/.

28. Neuman PJ, Chambers JD, Simon F, Meckley LM. Risk-sharing arrangements that link payment for drugs to health outcomes are proving hard to implement. *Health Affairs.* 2011;30(12):2329–2337. https://www .healthaffairs.org/doi/pdf/10.1377/hlthaff.2010.1147/.

29. Lucentis® (ranibizumab); abbreviated UK prescribing information. *Eye.* 2017;31:S18–S20. https://www.nature.com/articles/eye2017149/.

30. Technology appraisal guidance. Pegaptanib and ranibizumab for the treatment of age-related macular degeneration. National Institute for Health and Care Excellence. August 27, 2008; last updated May 1, 2012. https://www.nice.org.uk/guidance/ta155/resources/ranibizumab-and -pegaptanib-for-the-treatment-of-agerelated-macular-degeneration -82598316423109/.

31. Cigna press release. Cigna and Merck help customers better manage diabetes. Fierce Healthcare. October 28, 2010. https://www.fierce healthcare.com/healthcare/cigna-and-merck-help-customers-better -manage-diabetes/.

32. Numerof RE. Value added services: the second wave of disease management. Reuters Events: Pharma. June 19, 2014. https://www.reuters events.com/pharma/column/value-added-services-second-wave -disease-management/.

33. *Barriers to Value-Based Contracts for Innovative Medicines: PhRMA Member Survey Results.* STAT News. March 2017. https://www.statnews .com/wp-content/uploads/2017/03/PhRMA_ValueBased_Member Service_R2122-2.pdf.

34. Margolis Center for Health Policy. Value for Medical Products Consortium. https://healthpolicy.duke.edu/projects/value-medical-products -consortium/.

35. Value-Based Payment Advisory Group. Developing a path to value-based payment for medical products: background paper. April 28, 2017. https://healthpolicy.duke.edu/sites/default/files/2021-05/value _based_payment_background_paper_-_october_2017_final_0.pdf.

36. Novartis news release. Novartis receives first ever FDA approval for a CAR-T cell therapy, Kymriah™ (CTL019), for children and young adults with B-cell ALL that is refractory or has relapsed at least twice. August 30, 2017. https://www.novartis.com/news/media-releases/novartis -receives-first-ever-fda-approval-car-t-cell-therapy-kymriahm-ctl019

-children-and-young-adults-b-cell-all-refractory-or-has-relapsed-least-twice/.

37. Institute for Clinical and Economic Review. Chimeric antigen receptor T-cell therapy for cell cancers: effectiveness and value. Final Evidence Report. March 23, 2018. https://icer.org/wp-content/uploads/2020/10/ICER_CAR_T_Final_Evidence_Report_032318.pdf.

38. Spark Therapeutics press release. Spark Therapeutics announces first-of-their-kind programs to improve patient access to LUXTURNA™ (voretigene neparvovec-rzyl), a one-time gene therapy treatment. January 3, 2018. https://sparktx.com/press_releases/spark-therapeutics-announces-first-of-their-kind-programs-to-improve-patient-access-to-luxturna-voretigene-neparvovec-rzyl-a-one-time-gene-therapy-treatment/.

39. Alliance for Regenerative Medicine press release. ARM Foundation for Cell and Gene Medicine releases health economic impact landscape analysis led by IQVIA. August 6, 2018. https://alliancerm.org/press-release/arm-foundation-for-cell-and-gene-medicine-releases-health-economic-impact-landscape-analysis-led-by-iqvia/#.W2tcw1F7mRs.twitter/.

40. Cohen J. At over $2 million Zolgensma is the world's most expensive therapy, yet relatively cost-effective. *Forbes*. June 5, 2019. https://www.forbes.com/sites/joshuacohen/2019/06/05/at-over-2-million-zolgensma-is-the-worlds-most-expensive-therapy-yet-relatively-cost-effective/#e08b80245f5a/.

41. Marques Lopes J. Possible $4M price for AVXS-101, "foundational" SMA gene therapy, could be cost-effective, Novartis says. SMA News Today. November 9, 2018. https://smanewstoday.com/news-posts/2018/11/09/possible-4m-price-for-avxs-101-foundational-sma-gene-therapy-could-be-cost-effective-novartis-says/.

42. Walker J. Biotech proposes paying for pricey drugs by installment. *Wall Street Journal*. January 8, 2019. https://www.wsj.com/articles/biotech-proposes-paying-for-pricey-drugs-by-installment-11546952520/.

43. Liu A. Bluebird prices gene therapy Zynteglo at €1.575M in Europe, to be paid over 5 years. Fierce Pharma. June 14, 2019. https://www.fiercepharma.com/pharma/bluebird-prices-gene-therapy-zynteglo-at-eu1-575m-europe-to-be-paid-over-5-years/.

44. Daniel G, Leschly N, Marrazzo J, McClellan MB. Advancing gene therapies and curative health care through value-based payment reform. Health Affairs. October 30, 2017. https://www.healthaffairs.org/do/10.1377/hblog20171027.83602/full/.

45. Kolchinsky P, Brennan A, Karnal A, et al. Letter to President Biden, Secretary [of Health and Human Services] Xavier Becerra, [House] Speaker Nancy Pelosi, [Senate] Majority Leader Chuck Schumer, [House Republican] Leader Kevin McCarthy, [Senate Republican] Leader Mitch McConnell, America's lawmakers, patient advocates, and fellow Ameicans. September 8, 2021. https://global-uploads.webflow.com/606ac6e3ee6c271 3890937ef/61391fda6961aa750ebc2f1f_210908%20Affordability%20 and%20Innovation%20Letter.pdf.

chapter 11   Financial and Human Capital Investments in Biotechnology

1. Spector JM, Harrison RS, Fishman MC. Fundamental science behind today's important medicines. *Science Translational Medicine.* 2018; 10(438):eaaq1787.

2. DiMasi JA, Hansen RW, Grabowski HG. The price of innovation: new estimates of drug development costs. *Journal of Health Economics.* 2004; 22(2):151–185.

3. Forbes Live. *Healthcare Summit 2017: Five Fixes for Healthcare.* YouTube. December 1, 2017. https://www.youtube.com/watch?v=W1_PrpoA54 w&t=244s/.

4. National Human Genome Research Institute. Recombinant DNA (rDNA). https://www.genome.gov/genetics-glossary/Recombinant-DNA/.

5. Hughes SS. *Genentech: The Beginnings of Biotech.* University of Chicago Press; 2011.

6. Fraser L. Genentech goes public. Defining Moments. April 28, 2016. https://www.gene.com/stories/genentech-goes-public/.

7. Mukherjee S. *The Gene: An Intimate History.* Scribner; 2016.

8. Walters DKH. Genentech, Roche clear government hurdle to merger. *Los Angeles Times.* September 1, 1990. https://www.latimes.com/ar chives/la-xpm-1990-09-01-fi-299-story.html.

9. Pollack A. Roche agrees to buy Genetech for $46.8 billion. *New York Times.* March 12, 2009. https://www.nytimes.com/2009/03/13/busi ness/worldbusiness/13drugs.html?module=ArrowsNav&contentCol lection=Business%20Day&action=keypress&region=FixedLeft&pg type=article/.

10. Silicon Valley Bank. Healthcare investments & exits, annual 2022. https://www.svb.com/trends-insights/reports/healthcare-investments -and-exits#/.

11. Fincher D, director. *The Social Network.* Sony Pictures. 2010.

12. Pepitone J, Cowley S. Facebook's first big investor, Peter Thiel, cashes out. CNN Business. August 20, 2012. https://money.cnn.com/2012/08/20/technology/facebook-peter-thiel/index.html.

13. Wikipedia. Accel investment (Series A). The History of Facebook. https://en.wikipedia.org/wiki/History_of_Facebook#Accel_investment_(Series_A)/.

14. Levy A. Accel Facebook bet poised to become biggest venture profit: tech. Bloomberg. January 18, 2012. https://www.bloomberg.com/news/articles/2012-01-18/accel-s-facebook-bet-poised-to-become-biggest-ever-venture-profit-tech/.

15. Burnham B. Just how much did VC's pocket on Google? Burnham's Beat Blog. June 24, 2005. https://billburnham.blogs.com/burnhamsbeat/2005/06/just_how_much_d.html.

16. Booth BL, Salehizadeh B. In defense of life sciences venture investing. *Nature Biotechnology*. 2011;29(7):579–583.

17. Life Sci VC. Life sciences: the Rodney Dangerfield of venture capital. July 11, 2011. https://lifescivc.com/2011/07/life-sciences-the-rodney-dangerfield-of-venture-capital/.

18. Lalande K. Why venture capital doesn't scale. Santé Ventures White Paper v1.0. March 15, 2011. https://sante.com/wp-content/uploads/2020/05/Why-Venture-Doesnt-Scale-Sante-Ventures.pdf.

19. Life Sci VC. Framing up capital efficiency in early stage biotech. July 17, 2014. https://lifescivc.com/2014/07/framing-up-capital-efficiency-in-early-stage-biotech/.

20. Lewis M. *Moneyball: The Art of Winning an Unfair Game*. W. W. Norton; 2013.

21. Life Sci VC. VC-backed biotech ecosystem: a market in healthy equilibrium. March 10, 2017. https://lifescivc.com/2017/03/vc-backed-biotech-ecosystem-market-healthy-equilibrium/.

22. Bluestone JA, Deier D, Glimcher LH. The NIH is in danger of losing its edge in creating biomedical innovations. STAT News. January 3, 2018. https://www.statnews.com/2018/01/03/nih-biomedical-research-funding/.

23. Charette MF, Oh YS, Maric-Bilkan C, et al. Shifting demographics among research project grant awardees at the National Heart, Lung, and Blood Institute (NHLBI). *PLoS One*. 2016;11(12):e0168511. https://doi.org/10.1371/journal.pone.0168511/.

24. Herper M. Here, you can watch every second of the Forbes Healthcare Summit. *Forbes*. December 19, 2017. https://www.forbes.com/sites

/matthewherper/2017/12/19/here-you-can-watch-every-second-of
-the-forbes-healthcare-summit/#24a3b33f5720/.

25. Bill & Melinda Gates Foundation. JP Morgan Healthcare Conference.
January 8, 2018. https://www.gatesfoundation.org/ideas/Speeches
/2018/01/JP-Morgan-Healthcare-Conference/.

26. National Cancer Institute. The Cancer Genome Atlas program. https://
www.cancer.gov/about-nci/organization/ccg/research/structural
-genomics/tcga/.

27. US Food and Drug Administration. 21st Century Cures Act. January 31,
2020. https://www.fda.gov/regulatory-information/selected-amend
ments-fdc-act/21st-century-cures-act/.

28. Remarks by the president and the vice president at the 21st Century
Cures Act bill signing. Delivered at the South Court Auditorium.
Obama White House. December 13, 2016. https://obamawhitehouse
.archives.gov/the-press-office/2016/12/13/remarks-president-and
-vice-president-21st-century-cures-act-bill-signing/.

29. Gottleib S. *Submission to Congress: Food & Drug Administration Work
Plan and Proposed Funding Allocations of FDA Innovation Account.*
June 7, 2017. https://www.fda.gov/media/105635/download/.

30. Gottleib S. Implementing the 21st Century Cures Act: a 2018 update
from FDA and NIH. Testimony before the Subcommittee on Health, En-
ergy and Commerce Committee, US House of Representatives. July 24,
2018. https://www.fda.gov/NewsEvents/Testimony/ucm614607.htm.

31. US Food and Drug Administration news release. FDA approves first
cancer treatment for any solid tumor with a specific genetic feature.
May 23, 2017. https://www.fda.gov/news-events/press-announce
ments/fda-approves-first-cancer-treatment-any-solid-tumor-specific
-genetic-feature/.

32. Hudson KL, Collins FS. The 21st Century Cures Act—a view from the
NIH. *New England Journal of Medicine.* 2017;376(2):111–113.

33. Howard Hughes Medical Institute. History. https://www.hhmi.org
/about/history/.

34. Howard Hughes Medical Institute. Nobel lauteates. https://www.hhmi
.org/scientists/nobel-laureates/.

35. Bill & Melinda Gates Foundation. Our story. https://www.gatesfounda
tion.org/about/our-story/.

36. Bill & Melinda Gates Foundation. Foundation fact sheet. https://www
.gatesfoundation.org/about/foundation-fact-sheet/.

37. Bill & Melinda Gates Foundation. JP Morgan Healthcare Conference.

January 8, 2018. https://www.gatesfoundation.org/ideas/Speeches/2018
/01/JP-Morgan-Healthcare-Conference/.

38. Parker Institute for Cancer Immunotherapy at UCSF. University of California San Francisco. https://pici.ucsf.edu.

39. Chan Zuckerberg Initiative. Can we cure all diseases in our children's lifetime? September 21, 2016. https://chanzuckerberg.com/newsroom/can-we-cure-all-diseases-in-our-childrens-lifetime/.

40. Ortutay B. Zuckerberg, Chan pledge $3B to end disease. AP News. September 21, 2016. https://apnews.com/95af590f71cf4392b3b054ecc025
4c4a/zuckerbergs-have-new-charitable-goal-end-all-disease/.

41. Baltimore D. The boldness of philanthropists. *Science*. 2016;353(6307): 1473. https://www.science.org/doi/10.1126/science.aak9610/.

42. About Arc Institute. Arc Institute. https://arcinstitute.org/about/.

43. Piper K. Can a new approach to funding scientific research unlock innovation? Vox. December 18, 2021. https://www.vox.com/future-perfect
/2021/12/18/22838746/biomedicine-science-grants-arc-institute/.

chapter 12 **Looking Forward**

1. National Human Genome Research Institute. What is the Human Genome Project? October 28, 2018. https://www.genome.gov/12011238
/an-overview-of-the-human-genome-project/.

2. Venter JC, Adams MD, Myers EW, et al. The sequence of the human genome. *Science*. 2001;291(5507):1304–1351. https://science.sciencemag
.org/content/291/5507/1304/.

3. International Human Genome Sequencing Consortium. Initial sequencing and analysis of the human genome. *Nature*. 2001;409(6822):860–921.

4. Zimmer C. Scientists finish the human genome at last. *New York Times*. July 23, 2021. https://www.nytimes.com/2021/07/23/science/human
-genome-complete.html.

5. Nurk S, Koren S, Rhie A, et al. The complete sequence of a human genome. *bioRχiv*. May 27, 2021 [preprint]. https://www.biorxiv.org/con
tent/10.1101/2021.05.26.445798v1/.

6. Lappalainen T, MacArthur DG. From variant to function in human disease genetics. *Science*. 2021;373(6562):1464–1468.

7. National Human Genome Research Institute. DNA sequencing costs: data. https://www.genome.gov/27541954/dna-sequencing-costs-data/.

8. Moore's Law. How overall processing power for computers will double every two years. www.mooreslaw.org.

9. Fagan A. From 13 years to 20 hours, genome sequencing breaks record. GenomeMag.com. March 1, 2018. https://genomemag.com/2018/03/from-13-years-to-20-hours-genome-sequencing-breaks-record/.

10. Burke A. DNA sequencing is now improving faster than Moore's Law! *Forbes.* January 12, 2012. https://www.forbes.com/sites/techonomy/2012/01/12/dna-sequencing-is-now-improving-faster-than-moores-law/.

11. Rady Children's Hospital press release. New GUINNESS WORLD RECORDS™ title set for fastest genetic diagnosis. February 12, 2018. https://www.rchsd.org/about-us/newsroom/press-releases/new-guinness-world-records-title-set-for-fastest-genetic-diagnosis/.

12. Preston J, VanZeeland A, Peiffer DA. Innovation at Illumina: the road to the $600 human genome. Sponsor feature. *Nature Portfolio.* February 10, 2021. https://www.nature.com/articles/d42473-021-00030-9#:~:text=Today%2C%20a%20human%20genome%20can,study%20of%20diseases%20and%20phenotypes/.

13. Alliance for Regenerative Medicine. Record financing drives sector growth. ARM's Q3 2020 Trend Talk. https://alliancerm.org/sector-report/q3-2020-trend-talk/.

14. Office of Science Policy. Recombinant DNA Advisory Cmmittee archives. National Institutes of Health. https://osp.od.nih.gov/biotechnology/recombinant-dna-advisory-committee/.

15. Premier Research. Regulatory oversight on gene therapy in the U.S. and EU. March 8, 2019. https://premier-research.com/perspectives-regulatory-gene-therapy/.

16. Collins FS, Gottlieb S. The next phase of human gene-therapy oversight. *New England Journal of Medicine.* 2018;379(15):1393–1395. https://www.nejm.org/doi/10.1056/NEJMp1810628/.

17. US Food and Drug Administration. Cellular & gene therapy guidances. https://www.fda.gov/vaccines-blood-biologics/biologics-guidances/cellular-gene-therapy-guidances/.

18. US Food and Drug Administration statement. Statement from FDA Commissioner Scott Gottlieb, M.D. on agency's efforts to advance development of gene therapies. July 11, 2018. https://www.fda.gov/news-events/press-announcements/statement-fda-commissioner-scott-gottlieb-md-agencys-efforts-advance-development-gene-therapies/.

19. Marks P, Gottlieb S. Balancing safety and innovation for cell-based regenerative medicine. *New England Journal of Medicine.* 2018;378(10):954–959.

20. MIT NEWDIGS [NEW Drug Development ParadIGmS] Initiative. *FoCUS Project: Financing of Cures in the US*. November 2017. Research Brief 2017F211.v011. https://newdigs.mit.edu/sites/default/files/FoCUS _Research_Brief_2017F211v011.pdf.

21. Celgene press release. Updated results of ongoing multicenter Phase I study of bb2121 anti-BCMA CAR T cell therapy continue to demonstrate deep and durable responses in patients with late-stage relapsed/ refractory multiple myeloma at ASCO Annual Meeting. June 1, 2018. https://ir.celgene.com/press-releases-archive/press-release-details/2018 /Updated-Results-of-Ongoing-Multicenter-Phase-I-Study-of-bb2121 -anti-BCMA-CAR-T-Cell-Therapy-Continue-to-Demonstrate-Deep-and -Durable-Responses-in-Patients-with-Late-Stage-RelapsedRefractory -Multiple-Myeloma-at-ASCO-Annual-Meeting/default.aspx.

22. US Food and Drug Administration news release. FDA approves first cell-based gene therapy for adult patients with multiple myeloma. March 27, 2021. https://www.fda.gov/news-events/press-announcements/fda-ap proves-first-cell-based-gene-therapy-adult-patients-multiple-myeloma/.

23. Bristol-Myers Squibb press release. Bristol-Myers Squibb and bluebird bio announce positive top-line results from the pivotal Phase 2 KarMMa study of ide-cel in relapsed and refractory multiple myeloma. December 6, 2019. https://news.bms.com/news/details/2019/Bristol-Myers -Squibb-and-bluebird-bio-Announce-Positive-Top-line-Results-from -the-Pivotal-Phase-2-KarMMa-Study-of-Ide-cel-in-Relapsed-and-Re fractory-Multiple-Myeloma/default.aspx.

24. Tmunity Therapeutics. T cells hold the power to transform the treatment of devastating human diseases. https://www.tmunity.com.

25. Allogene Therapeutics. About us. https://www.linkedin.com/company /allogene-therapeutics/.

26. Sarepta Therapeutics press release. Sarepta Therapeutics anounces that at its first R&D Day, Jerry Mendell, M.D. presented positive preliminary results from the first three children dosed in the Phase 1/2a gene therapy micro-dystrophin trial to treat patients with Duchenne muscular dystrophy. June 19, 2018. https://investorrelations.sarepta.com/news -releases/news-release-details/sarepta-therapeutics-announces-its -first-rd-day-jerry-mendell-md/.

27. Collins F. Accelerating cures in the genomic age: the sickle cell example. NIH Director's Blog. December 11, 2018. https://directorsblog.nih.gov /2018/12/11/accelerating-cures-in-the-genomic-age-the-sickle-cell- example/.

28. Benz EJ Jr. The Cure Sickle Cell Initiative: catalyzing progress via innovative interfaces between NIH, patients, academics, ASH [American Society of Hematology], and the private sector. *Hematologist.* 2018; 15(6):9083. https://ashpublications.org/thehematologist/article/doi /10.1182/hem.V15.6.9083/463084/The-Cure-Sickle-Cell-Initiative -Catalyzing/.

29. Intellia Therapeutics press release. Intellia and Regeneron announce landmark clinical data showing deep reduction in disease-causing protein after single infusion of NTLA-2001, an investigational CRISPR therapy for transthyretin (ATTR) amyloidosis. June 28, 2021. https:// ir.intelliatx.com/news-releases/news-release-details/intellia-and-regen eron-announce-landmark-clinical-data-showing/.

30. Gillmore JD, Gane E, Taubel J, et al. CRISPR-Cas9 *in vivo* gene editing for transthyretin amyloidosis. *New England Journal of Medicine.* 2021; 385(18):493–502. https://www.nejm.org/doi/full/10.1056/NEJMoa 2107454/.

31. Isaacson W. *The Code Breaker: Jennifer Doudna, Gene Editing and the Future of the Human Race.* Simon & Schuster; 2021.

Epilogue: COVID-19

1. Weiss SR. Forty years with coronaviruses. *Journal of Experimental Medicine.* 2020;217(5):e20200537.

2. Zhong NS, Zheng BJ, Li YM, et al. Epidemiology and cause of severe acute respiratory syndrome (SARS) in Guangdong, People's Republic of China, in February, 2003. *Lancet.* 2003;362(9393):1353–1358.

3. Hijawi B, Abdallat M, Sayaydeh A, et al. Novel coronavirus infections in Jordan, April 2012: epidemiological findings from a retrospective investigation. *Eastern Mediterranean Health Journal.* 2013;19(Suppl 1):S12–S18.

4. Centers for Disease Control and Prevention. Middle East Resperatory Syndrome (MERS). August 2, 2019. https://www.cdc.gov/coronavirus /mers/about/index.html.

5. Gates B. Innovation for pandemics. *New England Journal of Medicine.* 2018;378(22):2057–2060.

6. Johns Hopkins University & Medicines. Coronavirus Resource Center: global map. https://coronavirus.jhu.edu/map.html.

7. Beigel JH, Tomashek KM, Dodd LE, et al. Remdesivir for the treatment of COVID-19—final report. *New England Journal of Medicine.* 2020; 383(19):1813–1826.

8. Letter from Denise M. Hinton, chief scientist, [US] Food and Drug Administration, to Ashley Rhoades, manager, Regulatory Affairs, Gilead Sciences. October 22, 2020. https://www.fda.gov/media/137564/down load/.

9. Kalil AC, Patterson TF, Mehta AK, et al. Barcitinib plus remdesivir for hospitalized adults with Covid-19. *New England Journal of Medicine.* 2021;384(9):795–807. https://www.nejm.org/doi/full/10.1056/NEJM oa2031994/.

10. Lilly investors news release. Baricitinib rceives emergency use authorization from the FDA for the treatment of hospitalized patients with COVID-19. November 19, 2020. https://investor.lilly.com/news-re leases/news-release-details/baricitinib-receives-emergency-use-au thorization-fda-treatment/.

11. The RECOVERY Collaborative Group. Dexamethasone in hospitalized patients with Covid-19. *New England Journal of Medicine.* 2021;384(8): 693–704. https://www.nejm.org/doi/10.1056/NEJMoa2021436/.

12. Cohn J. Chinese researchers reveal draft genome of virus implicated in Wuhan pneumonia outbreak. Science Insider: Asia/Pacific. January 11, 2020. https://www.science.org/content/article/chinese-researchers -reveal-draft-genome-virus-implicated-wuhan-pneumonia-outbreak/.

13. Chen P, Nirula A, Heller B, et al. SARS-CoV-2 neutralizing antibody LY-CoV555 in outpatients with Covid-19. *New England Journal of Medicine.* 2021;384(3):229–237. https://www.nejm.org/doi/10.1056/NEJM oa2029849/.

14. Regeneron investor & media news release. Regeneron's COVID-19 outpatient trial prospectively demonstrates that REGN-COV2 antibody cocktail significantly reduced virus levels and need for further medical attention. October 28, 2020. https://investor.regeneron.com/news-re leases/news-release-details/regenerons-covid-19-outpatient-trial-pro spectively-demonstrates/.

15. Regeneron investor & media news release. Regeneron's casirivimab and imdevimab antibody cocktail for COVID-19 is first combination therapy to receive FDA emergency use authorization. November 21, 2020. https://newsroom.regeneron.com/news-releases/news-release -details/regenerons-regen-cov2-first-antibody-cocktail-covid-19-re ceive/.

16. Lilly investors news release. Lilly's neutralizing antibody bamlanivimab (LY-CoV555) receives FDA emergency use authorization for the treatment of recently diagnosed COVID-19. November 3, 2020. https://in

vestor.lilly.com/news-releases/news-release-details/lillys-neutralizing
-antibody-bamlanivimab-ly-cov555-receives-fda/.

17. Immunization Agenda 2030: a global strategy to leave no one behind. April 1, 2020. http://www.immunizationagenda2030.org.

18. Levitt SD. Moncef Slaoui: "It's unfortunate that it takes a crisis for this to happen." Transcript of *People I (Mostly) Admire*. Podcast, episode 9. December 11, 2020. https://freakonomics.com/podcast/moncef-slaoui -its-unfortunate-that-it-takes-a-crisis-for-this-to-happen/.

19. Brenner S, Jacob F, Meselson M. An unstable intermediate carrying information from genes to ribosomes for protein synthesis. *Nature*. 1961; 190(4776):576–581.

20. Gros F, Hiatt H, Gilbert W, Kurland CG, Risebrough RW, Watson JD. Unstable ribonucleic acid revealed by pulse labelling of *Escherichia coli*. *Nature*. 1961;190(4776):581–585.

21. Karikó K, Buckstein M, Ni H, Weissman D. Suppression of RNA recognition by toll-like receptors: the impact of nucleoside modification and the evolutionary origin of RNA. *Immunity*. 2005;23(2):165–175.

22. Astellas news release. Astellas to acquire Ganymed Pharmaceuticals— acquisition would expand Astellas' oncology pipeline with antibody in late-stage. October 28, 2016. https://newsroom.astellas.us/2016-10-28 -Astellas-to-Acquire-Ganymed-Pharmaceuticals/.

23. BioNTech. Our vision. https://biontech.de/our-dna/vision/.

24. Pfizer press release. Pfizer outlines five-point plan to battle COVID-19. March 13, 2020. https://www.pfizer.com/news/press-release/press-re lease-detail/pfizer-outlines-five-point-plan-battle-covid-19/.

25. Pfizer press release. Pfizer and BioNTech to co-develop potential COVID-19 vaccine. March 17, 2020. https://www.pfizer.com/news /press-release/press-release-detail/pfizer-and-biontech-co-develop -potential-covid-19-vaccine/.

26. Pfizer press release. Pfizer and BioNTech announce further details on collaboration to accelerate global COVID-19 vaccine development. April 9, 2020. https://www.pfizer.com/news/press-release/press-re lease-detail/pfizer-and-biontech-announce-further-details-collabora tion/.

27. Pfizer press release. BioNTech and Pfizer announce regulatory approval from German authority Paul-Ehrlich-Institut to commence first clinical trial of COVID-19 vaccine candidates. April 22, 2020. https:// www.pfizer.com/news/press-release/press-release-detail/biontech _and_pfizer_announce_regulatory_approval_from_german_authority

_paul_ehrlich_institut_to_commence_first_clinical_trial_of_covid_19
_vaccine_candidates/.

28. Warren L, Manos PD, Ahfeldt T, et al. Highly efficient reprogramming to pluripotency and directed differentiation of human cells with synthetic modified mRNA. *Cell Stem Cell*. 2010;7(5):618–630.

29. Nobel Foundation. The Nobel Prize in Physiology or Medicine 2012 was awarded jointly to Sir John B. Gurdon and Shinya Yamanaka "for the discovery that mature cells can be reprogrammed to become pluripotent." 2012. https://www.nobelprize.org/prizes/medicine/2012/sum mary/.

30. Flagship Pioneering. Noubar Afeyan: founder & CEO. https://www.flag shippioneering.com/people/noubar-afeyan/.

31. Flagship Pioneering. Moderna. https://www.flagshippioneering.com /companies/moderna/.

32. Moderna press release. Moderna's work on a potential vaccine against COVID-19. March 16, 2020. https://www.sec.gov/Archives/edgar/data /1682852/000119312520074867/d884510dex991.htm.

33. Corbett KS, Edwards DK, Leist SR, et al. SARS-CoV-2 mRNA vaccine design enabled by prototype pathogen preparedness. *Nature*. 2020; 586(7830):567–571.

34. Graham BS. Rapid COVID-19 vaccine development. *Science*. 2020; 368(6494):945–946.

35. Moderna press release. Moderna announces positive interim Phase 1 data for its mRNA vaccine (mRNA-1273) against novel coronavirus. May 18, 2020. https://investors.modernatx.com/news/news-details /2020/Moderna-Announces-Positive-Interim-Phase-1-Data-for-its -mRNA-Vaccine-mRNA-1273-Against-Novel-Coronavirus-05-18-2020 /default.aspx.

36. Pfizer press release. Pfizer and BioNTech announce early positive data from an ongoing Phase 1/2 study of mRNA-based vaccine candidate against SARS-CoV-2. July 1, 2020. https://www.pfizer.com/news/press -release/press-release-detail/pfizer-and-biontech-announce-early-posi tive-data-ongoing/.

37. Pfizer press release. Pfizer and BioNTech choose lead mRNA vaccine candidate against COVID-19 and commence pivotal Phase 2/3 global study. July 27, 2020. https://www.pfizer.com/news/press-release/press -release-detail/pfizer-and-biontech-choose-lead-mrna-vaccine-candi date/.

38. Moderna press release. Moderna announces Phase 3 COVE study of

mRNA vaccine against COVID-19 (mRNA-1273) begins. July 27, 2020. https://investors.modernatx.com/news/news-details/2020/Moderna-Announces-Phase-3-COVE-Study-of-mRNA-Vaccine-Against-COVID-19-mRNA-1273-Begins-07-27-2020/default.aspx.

39. Moderna press release. Biopharma leaders unite to stand with science. September 8, 2020. https://investors.modernatx.com/news/news-details/2020/Biopharma-Leaders-Unite-to-Stand-with-Science-09-08-2020/default.aspx.

40. Pfizer press release. Pfizer and BioNTech propose expansion of pivotal COVID-19 vaccine trial. September 12, 2020. https://www.pfizer.com/news/press-release/press-release-detail/pfizer-and-biontech-propose-expansion-pivotal-covid-19/.

41. Tirrell M, Miller L. Moderna slows coronavirus vaccine trial enrollment to ensure minority representation, CEO says. CNBC. September 4, 2020. https://www.cnbc.com/2020/09/04/moderna-slows-coronavirus-vaccine-trial-t-to-ensure-minority-representation-ceo-says.html.

42. Shear MD. Politics, science and the remarkable race for a coronavirus vaccine. *New York Times.* November 22, 2020. https://www.nytimes.com/2020/11/21/us/politics/coronavirus-vaccine.html#click=https://t.co/fBwmaKqTy4/.

43. Pfizer press release. Pfizer and BioNTech announce vaccine candidate against COVID-19 achieved success in first interim analysis from Phase 3 study. November 9, 2020. https://www.pfizer.com/news/press-release/press-release-detail/pfizer-and-biontech-announce-vaccine-candidate-against/.

44. Moderna press release. Moderna's COVID-19 vaccine candidate meets its primary efficacy endpoint in the first interim analysis of the Phase 3 COVE study. November 16, 2020. https://investors.modernatx.com/news/news-details/2020/Modernas-COVID-19-Vaccine-Candidate-Meets-its-Primary-Efficacy-Endpoint-in-the-First-Interim-Analysis-of-the-Phase-3-COVE-Study-11-16-2020/default.aspx.

45. US Food and Drug Administration. 162nd Vaccines and Related Biological Products Advisory Committee (VRBPAC) Meeting: open public meeting. https://www.fda.gov/media/144859/download/.

46. STAT staff. FDA advisory panel endorses Pfizer/BioNTech Covid-19 vaccine. STAT News. December 10, 2020. https://www.statnews.com/2020/12/10/tracking-the-fda-advisory-panel-meeting-on-the-pfizer-biontech-covid-19-vaccine/.

47. US Food and Drug Administration. 163rd Vaccines and Related Biolog-

ical Products Advisory Committee (VRBPAC) Meeting: open public meeting. December 17, 2020. https://www.fda.gov/media/145466/down load/.

48. STAT staff. FDA advisory panel endorses Moderna's Covid-19 vaccine, clearing way for authorization. STAT News. December 17, 2020. https://www.statnews.com/2020/12/17/moderna-vaccine-fda-panel/.

49. Moderna. Storage & handling [of Moderna COVID-19 vaccine]. https://www.modernatx.com/covid19vaccine-eua/providers/storage-handling/.

50. Pfizer press release. Pfizer and BioNTech celebrate historic first authorization in the U.S. of vaccine to prevent COVID-19. December 11, 2020. https://www.pfizer.com/news/press-release/press-release-detail/pfizer -and-biontech-celebrate-historic-first-authorization/.

51. Moderna press release. Moderna announces FDA authorization of Moderna COVID-19 vaccine in U.S. December 18, 2020. https://inves tors.modernatx.com/news/news-details/2020/Moderna-Announces -FDA-Authorization-of-Moderna-COVID-19-Vaccine-in-U.S.-12-18 -2020/default.aspx.

Index